D0561077

"In her native Peru, Gabriela Wiener has a reputation as a gonzo journalist who takes an active role in whatever subject she investigates, which as often as not involves sex, and not the vanilla variety. In this collection, her first translated into English, we meet a notorious polygamous pornographer; go to 6&9, a Barcelona sex club; interview the cruel Lady Monique de Nemours, a world-class dominatrix; visit Vanessa, a member of the European community of Latin American trans sex workers; get a first-hand look at the perils of threesomes; and explore other topics a tad too risqué to even name in a family newspaper. Suffice to say, Wiener's free-wheeling style is hugely entertaining."

SARAH MURDOCH, *TORONTO STAR*

"Reading Gabriela Wiener is a joy. Over the years, her work has made me cry, laugh, hurt, and most importantly, dream. Her essays are daring, intimate, and honest, containing the self-awareness of a poet and the sharp focus of a marksman. I'd follow her anywhere."

DANIEL ALARCÓN,
AUTHOR OF *AT NIGHT WE WALK IN CIRCLES*

"One of the most interesting writers of this generation is Gabriela Wiener, a Peruvian journalist best known for her high-spirited explorations of female sexuality. . . . Wiener is witty and fast-paced; many of her experiences, sexual and otherwise, are hard-won, territories explored and sometimes conquered, despite her neurotic misgivings, with courage and aplomb. Part of her appeal lies in the fact that she sometimes writes about sexual topics that have not been well explored, especially by women, and a sense of incredulity is part of the pleasure of reading her work. 'Is she really going to do that?' the reader wonders. 'Is she really going to write (and so openly) about doing that?' And then she does, and there's a slight but perceptible shift in the world because she did."

LISA FETCHKO, *LOS ANGELES REVIEW OF BOOKS*

"With sizzling prose and journalistic attentiveness, Wiener honors the no-clothes rule. She exposes her readers to not only her body, but also to the neuroses, fears, and fantasies that come with it. True to the first-person style of gonzo journalism, each of Wiener's fifteen transgressive *crónicas* pull readers into penetrative commentaries on infidelity, abortion, and threesomes, not to mention the ever-elusory 'Ninja Squirt.' . . . *Sexographies* strikes the delicate balance between carnal and curious. . . . It [expands] the meaning of what pleasure in life can be, sexual or otherwise."

MADELINE DAY, *THE PARIS REVIEW*

"What Peruvian essayist and 'gonzo' journalist, Wiener, does in this collection is endlessly fascinating. Whether experiencing sexual subcultures or an ayahuasca trip, she uses herself as the point of departure to delve into the infinite manifestations of being human."

KEATON PATTERSON, BRAZOS BOOKSTORE (HOUSTON, TX),
BEST NONFICTION BOOKS OF 2018

"Gabriela Wiener is a Peruvian sex writer, and *Sexografías* is a book of her collected essays. However, she doesn't just stay on the carnal, and uses her explorations of egg donation, swingers parties, cruising, and squirting as channels into meditations on motherhood, death, and immigration, all while staying sharp and funny and wild."

ALEJANDRA OLIVA, REMEZCLA

GABRIELA WIENER

NINE MOONS

Translated from the Spanish by
Jessica Powell

RESTLESS BOOKS
BROOKLYN, NEW YORK

First published as *Nueve lunas* by Mondadori, Barcelona, 2009

First Restless Books hardcover edition May 2020

Hardcover ISBN: 9781632062239
Library of Congress Control Number: 2019944223

This book is supported in part by an award from
the National Endowment for the Arts.

This work has been published with a subsidy from the
Ministry of Culture and Sport of Spain.

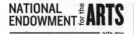

arts.gov

Cover design by Na Kim
Set in Garibaldi by Tetragon, London

Printed in Canada

1 3 5 7 9 10 8 6 4 2

Restless Books, Inc.
232 3rd Street, Suite A101
Brooklyn, NY 11215

www.restlessbooks.org
publisher@restlessbooks.org

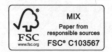

MIX
Paper from
responsible sources
FSC® C103567
www.fsc.org

For Elsi
For Lena

CONTENTS

NINE
MOONS

1

DECEMBER

OVER THESE PAST MONTHS, nine, to be exact, I've come to think that pleasure and pain always have something to do with things either entering or exiting your body.

Nine months ago I didn't know that a series of events related to those entrances and exits would converge that November, the same month I turned thirty. My father was diagnosed with colon cancer, Adriana committed suicide by throwing herself from a hotel window, and I was lying in a Spanish National Health Service hospital bed, recovering from major surgery. I returned home, devastated by the news, and physically very weak. I can scarcely remember the days following my operation, two weeks during a particularly cold winter, during which I'd needed J's help for almost everything. To cut my meat, to brush my teeth, and to clean my incisions.

I'd had some excess mammary glands removed from beneath my armpits and I could barely move my arms. I

3

had two enormous scars from which catheters emerged, draining dark blood. I'd decided to have the glands removed because, aside from being unattractive and annoying, the doctors had assured me that, one day in the remote future when I decided to have children, they would fill with milk and cause me terrible problems. And so I decided that I should amputate what I saw as a deformity, even though my mother, with her magical worldview, insisted on reminding me that in other times, women with supernumerary breasts were burned as witches: for her, my two extra breasts could have held supernatural powers.

The surgery went off without complications but the recovery was turning out to be very difficult. On top of that, the antibiotics they had prescribed to prevent infection seemed to be burning a hole in my stomach.

On J's birthday, just a few weeks later, I was still feeling so uncomfortable that I decided to stay home. I don't tend to miss my spouse's birthdays, so this was unusual. Now, in addition to intense stomach pain, I was nauseated. The next day, when it was time for me to go back to the office, I couldn't get out of bed. I was too tired. I threw up the entire morning. At noon, J called to see how I was doing, but also to give me some news.

"Don't panic. Okay? The magazine's closing. It's done."

My father's prognosis unknown.
My friend throwing herself into the void.
My mammary glands hacked off.
And now I had lost my job.

J came through the door with a pregnancy test in his hand. We'd been toying with the idea for a few months, in a perpetual *coitus interruptus*. The true vow, before the "I'll love and respect you forever" part, is: "I promise not to come inside you." It's the first promise that gets broken.

There's a secret rebellion, maybe a stupid one, but a rebellion nonetheless, against the adult world, or against anything, in never having a condom in the bedside table. I've always thought the hottest thing is that familiar scene when the lovers are just about to climax and something interrupts them. Cut short, what could have been a good orgasm becomes the best orgasm. No complete orgasm can exceed a perfectly incomplete one. Pulling out is like retiring at the peak of your career, like writing a masterful volume of short stories and then disappearing, like killing yourself at the age of thirty.

We fell silent for a few seconds looking at the indicator; it's like looking at the gun you're going to use to kill yourself. A pregnancy test is always an intimidating presence, especially if you're freshly unemployed.

I had to pee in a vial, sprinkle a few drops on that white thingy while J read the instructions and finally figured out that two stripes means yes and one stripe means no. According to the box, a home pregnancy test is 99 percent accurate if the result is positive, while, if it's negative, there's a greater margin of error and the test should be repeated in a few days. I don't know how many times I'd taken that test in my life, the result almost always negative.

Women play all the time with the great power that has been conferred upon us: it's fun to think about reproducing. Or not reproducing. Or walking around in a sweet little dress with a round belly underneath that will turn into a baby to cuddle and spoil. When you're fifteen, the idea is fascinating, it attracts you like a piece of chocolate cake. When you're thirty, the possibility attracts you like an abyss.

On the leaflet it also said that pregnancy tests measure the presence in urine of a hormone called Human Chorionic Gonadotropin. This hormone, let's call it by its first name, Gona, appears in the blood approximately six days after conception, when the fertilized egg implants in the uterus. In the five minutes it took the gadget to decide what would become of my life, I scrolled in slow motion through every time I'd made love during the past month, trying to identify the fatal day. Finally, the two red bars quickly appeared, like the words "The End" in a movie.

"That's the last time we ever work together at the same place," I said to J.

Because now we could actually say that an entire family was about to be out on its ass, and facing the coldest Christmas in years, according to the weatherman. Although the weatherman is usually wrong.

Two gametes form a zygote. I like the way the fertilization formula sounds. It's pure math. The most powerful feelings upon discovering that you're pregnant have to do with the unreality of the math. They've told you it's there, that it will multiply in size, that now it's the shape of a peanut, and then a cherry, and so on, but you don't see it, you don't feel it. I could have opted to pay two hundred euros for one of those ultramodern sonogram machines that show you what's inside, but for now, I would limit myself to consulting direct testimonies. To one woman, a four-week-old embryo looked like a shrimp, to another, it was a pea, to another, a little fish, and to another, a spot in the distance. Why should maternity draw us immediately into lyrical digressions and take us to the edge of inanity? Could the mere possibility of having a baby with the face of a frightened monkey in our arms be enough to trigger that unbridled tenderness? I decided to write my own zoological turn of phrase: "At four weeks, a child is like the ghost of a seahorse."

The truth is you still can't see anything. Just the premature gestational sac, less than ten centimeters in diameter, the bag inside which the fetus will grow. What an awful word "fetus" is. It's so ugly. An embryo looks like something that could only be aquatic. It doesn't look human. It has a tail. It's four millimeters long and its eyes are like the pair of black dots that you sometimes find in a raw egg before putting it in the skillet.

In my old encyclopedia of the human body, I read that in an embryo you can already make out the spinal column, the lungs and the rest of the organs, all on a minuscule scale. However, a four-week-old baby is not a human being, it's hundreds of species all at once. Up until recent decades, it was thought that the human baby passed through every stage of evolution inside the mother's womb, that it had the gills of a fish and the tail of a monkey. It seemed plausible. Then it was proven that those weren't really gills and that wasn't really a tail, but, in seeing the images of a fetus's evolution, one might well conclude that pregnancy is the trailer for the movie of life. Would you like to see the whole film?

Books don't prepare you for what's coming. Manuals for pregnant women must have been written by mothers completely drugged by love for their children, without the slightest pinch of critical distance. They all say: you'll feel slight nausea in the morning, your breasts will become full and tender, you'll feel tired and the frequent need to urinate. Ah, and of course: "don't smoke, don't drink coffee or Coca-Cola, don't take drugs, avoid X-rays." How the hell am I supposed to bear all this stress without even a can of Coca-Cola? How is it that no one has yet created a designer drug for pregnant women? Prenatal ecstasy, LSD for expectant mothers, something like that.

To start with, it's not just nausea; the fundamental malaise that seizes you when you wake up in the morning is like waking up with a hangover and a guilty conscience all at the same time, like waking up after a loved one's funeral or seeing dawn break on the day after losing the love of your life. The nausea would attack me in the most inopportune places and times. I started to think that it revealed a certain psychology in my relationship with things. For example, I always got nauseated when I had to do something that I didn't want to do, like go out to buy bread very early in the morning in the middle of winter. It also appeared when I was with a certain, very beloved friend. Every time I saw her I would have to run to the bathroom.

Don't even get me started on my breasts; they hurt at the slightest touch. They weren't the only sensitive things. It was all of me. I never imagined that I could cry watching one of those horrendous talk shows hosted by some snake in the grass who interviews children searching for their mothers and neighbors who hate each other; but cry I did, oceans of tears, especially at stories like: "Her husband cheated on her with the ninety-nine-cent-store clerk. . . . Let's bring out the huuuuusband!" I, a person with advanced degrees, raised in a home where we listened to Silvio Rodríguez and Quilapayún, would find myself curled in a fetal position under a blanket, the remote control my only umbilical cord to the world. And someone had pressed the slow-motion button.

I spent long hours watching trash TV, sleeping and dreaming that I was giving birth to a monkey.

My sister and I had a game. We would announce: "Let's play mother and daughter." We were always mothers and we were always mothers to daughters. The maternal world was a world for women alone. It was very easy to be a mother: it consisted of naming our dolls, covering them with a blanket, and combing their hair. And when I was the scriptwriter, some sort of tragedy always had to occur, a devastating earthquake, for example, that would infuse a little drama into the maternal role. Our dolls would cry and we would protect them from the hurricane-force winds and take them somewhere safe. It was lovely to be a mother when we were in danger. It made us better mothers.

Barcelona seemed like a good place for two naive journal-ists with literary aspirations who believed in the possibili-ties of their résumés, but not for two aspiring journalists with a child. J and I had gone to work for the magazine *Lateral*, first for nothing and then for very little. But we were happy to be able to dedicate ourselves to our vocations after working various jobs invented to exploit undocumented immigrants. We hadn't arrived on a raft, but our status as foreign students relegated us to the lowest rung on the employment ladder.

No one here cares what you might have done before in some place in the southern hemisphere. Your self-published little books are worthless. Ditto that preten-tious-sounding master's degree you've come here to com-plete. It won't do you any good to say you were published in the most important media outlets in your country and that you won a prize.

That's why you'll end up working for free like the oldest intern known to man. Your thirties aren't exactly the most auspicious runway for launching your career.

On top of that, they speak Catalan in this city and the Catalans want us to speak to them in their language, even though they are perfectly bilingual, so they tend to offer the good jobs to those who speak it. The Catalans are super nice about a lot of things, but when it comes to the topic of language, they're total drags.

And even though you know nothing about it, you'll try to earn money in the prosperous restaurant world as a waitress serving seafood paella. You'll work for speculators during the real estate bubble, selling off apartments that had belonged to evicted little old ladies. You'll deliver junk mail door to door, risking being bitten by a ferocious dog, or you'll be a voice on the telephone selling whatever.

The good thing about Barcelona is they celebrate a cute holiday during which people exchange books and roses. It's sort of like Valentine's Day but instead of going to the movies, couples go shopping at bookstores. This gives you the sense—not always correct—that you're surrounded by sensitive, cultured people. Here, the newsstands on La Rambla, bulging with newspapers and magazines, look like supermarket shelves. Here, people read on the metro, though later you realize they're reading Coelho and Dan Brown. Here, the local soccer team always wins. And, like it or not, that winning spirit is contagious.

Maybe all of this is why it was actually enjoyable to allow myself to be exploited by a literary publication run by people as fun and learned as *Lateral*'s director, Mihály Dés, a Hungarian-born Jewish intellectual who had settled in Spain many years back; and its editor in chief, Robert Juan-Cantavella, the youngest, most handsome, most rock-star boss one could ever dream of. Mihály had become an entrepreneur in order to pursue the dream of running an independent journal and he'd done the impossible in keeping it afloat for eleven years. But debt had sunk it in the end. At least, just before it went under completely, taking advantage of the massive regularization of immigrants the government was undertaking, J and I had managed to get *Lateral* to extend us an employment contract, our very first in Spain. In this way, we had changed our status from students to residents with legal employment. But we had to find other jobs right away or we would lose our precarious legal status.

What would we do with a child outside of Peru? Would we dress him in clothing from a dumpster, make him live with five drunken students, get him a Barça membership card? Certainly we would tell him that a person's dignity isn't defined by one's job. We'd teach him not to take taxis because they're very expensive and to ride his bike in the rain. On Sundays we'd take him to IKEA. Or better yet, we'd train him to do a weekly search through the trash for almost-new household appliances. We'd buy him clothes at Humana, that chain of second-hand clothing stores run by people who care about the environment. We'd take him to do our weekly grocery shopping at Día, the run-down supermarket where the carts of derelicts, squatters and neglected retirees clash in the aisles. And if all that weren't convincing enough, we'd tell him that he'd always be able to drink coffee and eat croissants while leafing through *El País* on a crowded, sun-dappled terrace at midday, while others were busy busting their humps. And that he should read Henry Miller. My child: Europe is the best place for a Latin American to starve to death and drink good wine. Welcome.

When I went down to take out the trash, I picked up a free newspaper and, by chance, found myself looking at a typical headline about immigration: "Fifteen percent of people born in Spain are the children of immigrants." That's how we are, we jump into bed so enthusiastically that we end up balancing the demographic scales in a country with the lowest birth rate in the world. It's only thanks to us that there are more births in Spain than there are deaths. But a bit lower I read another headline in small print: "One third of abortions in Spain are sought by immigrants." In the article, a doctor declared that he treated many South American women who arrived bleeding to death "because they took aspirin and parsley." Does that work?

My first visit to the obstetrician, instead of making the news feel official, made everything seem even more unreal. Public insurance doesn't include such perks as ultrasounds every time you're in the mood to give your embryo a little tickle. Here, unlike in Lima, there's no Women's Diagnostic Center next to every no-tell motel. And so I was forced to wait until February for my first ultrasound, the first-trimester ultrasound. I'd have to live with it. The only clear news about this child had been delivered to me in the form of two red lines. I was going to spend Christmas and ring in the New Year without seeing so I could believe.

The purpose of that first visit was to establish contact with the midwife, the person monitoring the pregnant woman from month to month. There are only three scheduled visits with the gynecologist before the birth. The midwife is not a doctor but she knows everything about pregnant women and babies. They are the hospital versions of the self-taught neighbor ladies from other eras who would come to attend to you at home and cut through the umbilical cord with their teeth.

Eulalia appeared with her short, curly gray hair, her dirty white coat, and those inexplicable red high-heeled shoes that she always wore without stockings. She invited me in and, adjusting her thick glasses, prepared to take down my medical history. She gave me a little purple notebook that said *Carnet de l'embarassada*.

"Do you have a family history of cardiovascular disease, cancer, congenital defects, multiple pregnancies . . . ?"

My grandmother had been diabetic, my father had had a section of his intestine removed, several relatives had died of heart attacks, my great aunt had died of breast cancer. With her quasi-doctor's handwriting, Eulalia made note of some of the saddest parts of my biography, in the same style she probably used to make a grocery list. When we came to my own history, I mentioned my recently excised supernumerary glands and a cyst I'd had removed from my right ovary a few years back. Also three abortions. I felt a bit worse for wear.

"What's your LMP?"

"My . . . LMP?"

"Yes, your Last Menstrual Period."

I told her I didn't know when my LMP had been. I've always hated that moment when, just before inserting an apparatus to sound the depths of my insides (an apparatus that looks dangerously similar to an industrial orange juicer), the gynecologist asks about my last period. Because at the instant they ask me about it, I draw a complete blank. Over time, I decided not to admit that I couldn't remember, and from then on, I always said "the eleventh," which is my lucky number. She took out a cardboard wheel and began to fiddle with it in order to calculate what week of gestation I was in and the probable due date. Your little cabbage, she said, will be born in August. The word "cabbage" activated my own memories of the popular dolls, "Cabbage Patch Kids," that I'd had when I was a little girl. The song from the commercial was very cruel: "Cabbage Patch Kids were born from a flower/ Who will take care of them?/They have no mommy." And so a six-year-old girl got emotionally blackmailed into adopting a baby with a plastic head and a cloth body that their mom and dad would pay for.

"Lie down here, please."

I lay down on the exam table. Eulalia—who, I was later surprised to find out, was a gospel singer in addition to being a midwife—raised my T-shirt and began to prod my belly, which looked the same as always.

"Now we'll listen to its heart."

I would finally be able to confirm that something alive, something that wasn't my own soul, was inhabiting me. She put an ultrasound monitor on my belly. At first, the silence was absolute. Eulalia moved the wand from side to side and I started to think that I was maybe some sort of crazy lady with one of those imaginary pregnancies. Until, at last, the exam room filled with an outrageous "boom boom."

"That's its heartbeat."

". . ."

"And this one is yours."

The difference in rhythm was shocking. A fetal heart beats at a rate of 120 to 160 beats per minute, while an adult heart beats only 76 times per minute. The heart of a fetus is, proportionally, more than nine times bigger than a full-grown human's. From the eighteenth day onward, it beats and beats without stopping until the moment of our death. The sound of that muscle is almost the first human manifestation. Once upon a time, we too were only a heartbeat. Only much later do we become bigger than our hearts.

When I left the office, I read in *My Baby and Me*, the magazine Eulalia had just subscribed me to, that this Christmas, among all the iPods and MP3 players, there was also a gadget that uses Doppler technology to listen to the fetal heartbeat inside a mother's belly. "Without having to go to the doctor," said the advertisement, and "using a cable hookup," you can record the sounds or connect a telephone to share them with others: for only 69 euros, "we can also feel its little kicks, when it has the hiccups, and even record the mother's heartbeat to calm the baby after it's born."

Soon we'll be able to chat with our fetus in real time.

When I got home, I wrote in my blog: "Its heart beats like a sampler from a mentally unstable DJ; its heart is pure electronica while mine is an old progressive rock song."

There comes a time in life when a woman has to recognize that she's no longer able to write the sexual autobiography of a Lolita. After all the memoirs of fiery Italian girls and adolescent Chinese S&M aficionados that I'd come across, I'd established that there's an age limit for scandal. Or maybe not. In any case, I didn't feel like making a fool of myself for such little money and with no guarantee that I'd become a best-selling author, or at least a Catherine Millet, the French art critic who recounted how she got banged by a whole pack of guys in the middle of a forest, among other intimacies. There are times when one should take life more seriously than literature. Not many, but they do exist.

Shortly after I arrived in Barcelona, I was hired by *Primera Línea*, a magazine that, in the 80s, had been one of the artifacts of cultural disinhibition and among those that most quickly acceded to the changing mores of the times. In sum: it was a pioneer when it came to publishing tits on its covers. My boss, Guillermo Hernaiz, is the only authentic hedonist I've ever known. Guillermo organizes fetish and DJ parties at the most popular clubs, and he always has an over-the-top assignment for me. I'm his favorite gonzo journalist, his kamikaze, as he likes to call me. Under the pseudonym Ada Franela, I've written the most sensationalized pieces in every issue. For one of them, I allowed myself to be whipped by a bloodthirsty dominatrix in front of a packed auditorium, before becoming her apprentice. For stories like that one, I got interviewed on the radio and on television. A couple of pieces for *PL* paid almost the same as *Lateral* paid me for a whole month of work. Writing about sex had become profitable. As it happens, just as I found out that I was expecting a baby, I was putting the finishing touches on a book.

It had started as a piece of investigative journalism, transformed instead into a gonzo chronicle, and ended finally as a testimonial with the trappings of a questionable erotic novel. Immediately after reading the piece I wrote for the magazine *Etiqueta Negra* about liberal-minded people who derive sexual pleasure from swapping partners, the editor of *Primera Línea* offered me work. But the next gift bestowed by the swingers tribe would be that a publishing house would commission me to write a tell-all book about that subculture. In the last few months, I had dedicated myself, along with J, to visiting liberal clubs and parties, participating in orgies and even promoting them among our acquaintances. In addition to this rigorous fieldwork, I had gotten my hands on a copious bibliography—from Boccaccio to Bataille, through to Melissa P.—that was piling up on my desk.

Was it right that this tiny cell would one day learn to read? When he asks me where babies come from, would I encourage him to look on the bookshelf for his mother's erotic confessions? How does one raise a human being to be able to cope with his childhood friends' jeers about his mother's technical descriptions of group sex? In which alternative high school should I enroll him?

Alongside the pile of books about sexual perversions, a separate tower composed of maternity handbooks, month-by-month pregnancy guides, and psychology texts for first-time mothers was taking shape.

My last piece for *Primera Línea* was an article called "Do You Want to Have Sex With Me?" It was about fictitiously proposing sex to all sorts of men, and recording their reactions. I stationed myself at midnight in the doorway to the bathroom at a disco called Fellini to offer myself to every man who passed by. A large number of them responded that they never had sex on the first date. When I got home, I wrote that you had to woo the men of today with flowers and chocolates. I was one month pregnant.

Virginia Woolf didn't have children. Neither did Eva Perón. How was I ever going to become a household name now that I had turned into a regurgitant being? The poetry of Sylvia Plath, one of my favorite poets, had improved greatly after she had her children, but soon after, she had killed herself by turning on the gas and sticking her head in the oven. I wasn't interested in paying such a high price to be a good writer. To begin with, pregnancy turns you into a bag of gases. There's not a shred of poetry in that, I can assure you.

Every day I told J that if we had any doubts at all we still had time to end this thing. I asked myself if it would be equally valid to write my own *Letter to a Child Never Born*, Oriana Fallaci's epistolary novel, if I had to add: "because of my own fault." How could I help but read that slim volume during those hours of unhealthy hesitation? I discovered that Oriana, the now hyper-conservative Italian writer known for her anti-Islamic fascism and her declared homophobia, was also capable of crafting a lovely metaphor when she discovered she was pregnant. She said: "You seemed like a mysterious flower, a transparent orchid." Everyone, a murderer, a rapist of children, the president of a superpower, we all discover the poet inside us upon imagining "that drop of life that escaped from nothingness." Anyway, like Fallaci but in a different way, I could explain sweetly and pedagogically to my fetus that abortion is an inalienable right of emancipated women. I would write: "Dear embryo, you are only a mammalian blueprint, ignorant of the power that others have over your existence, you have no face, and even less a brain with which to sense my suspicious movements on the outside. Why would I pluck you from nothingness only to return you to nothingness?"

When I was twelve years old I saw my mother reading *The Second Sex* by the French feminist Simone de Beauvoir. The title had that three-letter word in it, so it must have contained something good. Also, I had never seen my mother keep a book with her for so long, the way other people carry the Bible under their arms. Yes, that book was my mother's Bible. It was worn and underlined, filled with small secret annotations. One day I finally stole it from her. I read it and it made such an impression on me that I came up with the idea of bringing it to school. I remember that, before the start of class, I read out loud to my girlfriends entire paragraphs about the necessity of resisting our biological destiny. For Beauvoir, women passively suffered that destiny, doing household chores, reconciling themselves to maternity. For her, bearing children and breastfeeding did not imply any sort of life plan, they were natural and imposed functions. But in the afternoons, my boyfriend would pick me up from school and we'd seek out some secluded place where I could surrender to my dark destiny as a woman.

Why the obsession with motherhood? As I write this, thousands of women are trying to procreate in every single place on the planet. With sperm banks, surrogate mothers, donated eggs. I know because I, myself, while I was writing a piece about egg donation, went to the Dexeus Clinic in Barcelona and donated ten of my eggs to an anonymous woman who couldn't get pregnant. And at this very moment, many other women are allowing the possibility to go down the drain.

I know that reproductive technologies will not stop until we can all become mothers. I'm writing about my pregnancy at the same moment in which people in white coats are conducting research into the possibility of female auto-procreation, male pregnancy, the gestation of human beings in animals and in women who are clinically dead.

I read this in a popular-science article: a child can be born with the genetic material of a third person whose identity he will never know. Twins can be born separated by several years. A woman can give birth to a baby she didn't conceive or that she conceived with the sperm of a dead man. A child can have up to five progenitors (ovular, gestational, social mother; genetic, social father). A grandmother can gestate a child conceived by her daughter and son-in-law. And even more spine-chilling is the fact that there are companies that sell reproductive services and women's body parts, like eggs and uteruses. Other companies specialize in the predetermination of fetal sex, like in India, where, I've read, 29 of every 30 female fetuses are aborted.

The same thing always happens to me around scientific advances: I don't know whether to laugh or to cry. Stories like the one I read in Élisabeth Roudinesco's book *The Family in Disorder* make me feel like I should get myself baptized: "In June 2001, the story of Jeanine Salomone, a native of Draguignan, was the talk of the town. At the age of sixty-two and after twenty unsuccessful attempts, she gave birth to a boy, Benoit-David, conceived with purchased eggs and the semen of her own brother, Robert, who was blind and paraplegic as a result of a suicide attempt involving a gun. She had introduced him as her husband and the

Californian doctor who pulled off the heroic feat didn't ask any questions about the couple's strange appearance. What's more, since the procedure produced an extra embryo, he implanted it in the uterus of a paid surrogate mother, who gave birth to Marie Cécile, born three weeks after Benoit-David. Adopted by Jeanine, the two children were, simultaneously, siblings, half siblings and cousins, and under no circumstances could they become the legal son and daughter of an incestuous couple. So, on the civil registry, they were simply recorded as the children of a celibate mother and an unknown father."

This was happening all around us. And I was simply pregnant. Not so much because I had wanted to be. To use a cliché: with the way the world is, one can't afford the luxury of wanting something too much. These days, a woman gets pregnant because the idea doesn't disgust her. Though it does make her a bit queasy.

2

JANUARY

It's not like I buried her under the patio.

PREGNANCY MANUALS have a lot to say about how to eat right, avoid smoking, and stay away from alcohol, about exercise and the fight against stretch marks, but not one of them says a thing about Rotten.com. Not one of them says: Stay away! Danger! You'll regret it. The site is an archive of macabre data and images. It specializes in horror in its most unbearable forms: coprophagia, dismemberment, autopsies, suicides, executions, massacres, celebrity deaths. . . . The alleged photo of Marilyn Monroe's corpse and the hanging of Saddam Hussein are there. But the most disturbing are the anonymous dead. I remembered browsing through the site in disgust a few years back, but in the days that followed the revelations of the pregnancy test, I went back to face the grim reaper who welcomes you to the Web. I don't know if it was the Molotov cocktail of hormones, but that "fantastical adventure called pregnancy," "the most thrilling wait of your life," "those nine unforgettable months," had unleashed my darkest of dark sides. I wasn't alone in this; I'd heard about pregnant women who couldn't stop imagining their babies with malformations. The bogeyman stalked them. They closed their eyes and saw their babies with deformities.

On Rotten, I succumbed to an irresistible link. It said: "The Ultimate Taboo." The Internet can transport you from one feeling to another, abysmally different feeling, in a single click. You're checking your email after peeling a tangerine and you come face to face with an impossible image:

A man is eating a baby.

A fried baby.

I don't know if the man was a criminal, a dinner guest with bizarre table manners, or an appalling prankster with a talent for Plasticine gore, but he was gobbling a small, golden child on a plate, eating its small arm like a crispy chicken wing. It looked way too real. It was real. And it was the first time that I felt like a lady. Or a person. Or a draft proposal for a mother with a draft proposal for morality. And it was the first time that I vomited like a true more-sensitive-than-most pregnant woman.

But I didn't vomit up my baby. In order to do that, I would have had to swallow him first. Like Saturn. Now that I think about it, that image on Rotten could well have been an homage to the Rubens painting hanging in the Prado in Madrid. For pure realism, it's even worse than Goya's. On the canvas, the god, Saturn, is eating one of his sons, chubby and blond like a cherub. He rips his chest apart with a single bite. The baby bleeds, its face agonizing. The Greek myth says that Saturn devoured his children because an oracle warned him that one of them would dethrone him. And that's what happened. Zeus was saved because his mother, Rhea, swapped him for a rock she wrapped in swaddling clothes. Then Zeus caused Saturn to vomit up his siblings.

That whole Freudian totemic banquet business made sense to me in those moments: eating the father for lunch is the ritual that symbolizes the culmination of the desire to take his place at the head of the tribe. The selfish father who wants all the females for himself expels his son from the cave, the son comes back with some friends, kills him and devours him. I expect that primitive humans allowed themselves to be cannibals when they were hungry. They didn't psychoanalyze it overmuch.

I was beginning to be devoured. There was no doubt about it. From the inside out. An umbilical cord had been created and, through it, the scrawny being was nourishing itself with the chemical substances that would make it grow fat. As a consequence, I had lost a little weight and I was anemic. I was its breakfast, lunch, and dinner. Its ten-euro weekday supper and its weekend feast. I took iron supplements and folic acid to bolster my hemoglobin levels. But the baby just went right on gobbling up all of my red blood cells. Using my nutrients, a placenta had formed, a sac that protected the fetus, even from me, a kind of squishy armchair where it would rest as it waited to become a fetus.

At that moment, more than anything else, my small inhabitant seemed like a tumor. Its cells rapidly grew and multiplied, penetrating my tissues and eroding my blood vessels. It was a parasite that lived off my expense, extracting its strength and nourishment from my body. It breathed my oxygen. And I panted.

While the tiny tadpole struggled to bind itself to life, I was thinking that we were headed straight for disaster. My future, and J's, hung by a thread. We had two airplane tickets—Barcelona–Madrid–Lima/Lima–Madrid–Barcelona—for the end of February. We had bought them several months ahead of time, not knowing that the magazine was going to go under. What could have been a cause for rejoicing, the longed-for visit after two years of absence now seemed like a bad idea. The planned trip had several disadvantages. In Lima, we were sure to spend a large portion of the money we had saved and that would leave us in a very vulnerable situation when we returned, especially now that we were unemployed. By the time we got back, it was likely I'd be showing, and then who would want to hire a pregnant woman who would only grow fatter and more tired, who would soon have to leave work because of excessive weight? The day would come when I'd have to run off to the hospital and then disappear for four months, the duration of maternity leave. And anyway, I would no longer be able to produce the same daring stories at the same pace as before. And at some point, I had to admit, I wouldn't be able to produce anything. Except, probably, milk. What some people saw as a promising journalistic career was being cut short and there was no way to stop the losing streak.

J, for his part, had started working in the telemarketing department of a company that offered no-interest credit cards. J didn't turn his nose up at any sort of work. And anyway, it was very good for us to have some money coming in so we wouldn't go completely broke. I had also sent out some résumés but no one had called me, so I spent all day alone at home. I didn't even feel like writing because I had just finished the book about swingers. I felt a little bit embarrassed to have so much free time. But I also lacked energy. I was wrecked by nausea. They say that the nausea is a response to the emotional black hole that comes with the knowledge that you're going to be a mother.

At two months of pregnancy, the baby is completely formed. It has an enormous mouth, a squashed nose and still lidless eyes, open to the most unfathomable darkness. The "your baby, month by month" guides describe in such minute detail the development of their facial features, their extremities, their digestive and nervous systems, that by afternoon, my compassion for those little arms lined with blue and red veins overwhelmed me completely, as did my urge to hug that poor little embryo and knit it a scarf for its innocent little tail.

But as night fell, darker thoughts overtook me. The vast majority of abortions are done at that stage, in the second month, when its presence can be easily detected: it makes it very easy to catch that little fish in the net. Its joints still have the flexibility of cartilage. After two months it's dangerous because the baby's bones have hardened and can damage the walls of the uterus. While the manuals softened me up, Google continued to supply the sinister imagery that my state of mind demanded. "Abortion at two months," I typed, and photos that could easily have appeared on Rotten.com popped up. In one photo, you could see a tiny, perfectly formed arm, as big around as a toothpick, torn off and bleeding. The photo had clearly been doctored. The arm of an eight-week old embryo can't be that size, when its entire body measures two centimeters at most. Although its shape is human, you need a microscope to see it.

The embryo activates a hormone in the mother to prevent the rejection that naturally occurs in the body when faced with the presence of an invader. I sensed that the nausea was my body's reaction to an unidentified foreign object. Like when you take a drug and you feel a bit queasy or like you have to go to the bathroom. Our immune systems detect the presence of the enemy and struggle to expel it. Our bodies are capable of employing the most lethal methods to be rid of the intruders. If, upon implanting in the uterus, the future baby didn't send out signals so as not to be confused for a foreign body, it would be destroyed by its own mother. But, apparently, sometimes the mother doesn't understand the language of hormones and/or she ignores the message. Or she simply presses delete.

According to anti-abortion manifestos, an embryo feels pain, "it violently resists being dismembered alive." I can't help but feel like a serial killer. Only a woman who has had an abortion knows what it means. The reprimand can come from outside and from within one's own self. There are always people prowling about, laws, priests, moral precepts, telling us why we should suffer or why we shouldn't. Is the question really when does life begin? At conception, in the first week or in the twenty-eighth, or when it's an egg containing DNA or a fetus that can live outside the uterus, when it's a newborn or a child raised among humans? The writer, Hernán Migoya, posted in a blog that he was in favor of "postpartum abortion," now that all of his friends were having children and he was not. He argued that he would never have children because he was his own child: "I couldn't bear the thought that a child would displace me from the center of attention, be it from someone else's or, worse, from my own! I don't know what the fuck people are thinking when they have kids. They want to give up being the center of their own lives just like that? Are they so eager to be free of themselves?" Migoya says that all artists have been horrendous parents, real sons of bitches as parents. And what if the murderous instinct should awaken much later? How many ways are there to kill in a lifetime? Who condemns those crimes?

Women who have had an abortion live through their own pain and mourning in silence. How great it would be if regret and guilt and pain could be vacuumed up and tossed in a bin. But that isn't possible.

I remembered that J had told me about a horror film from the 70s that could very easily have been produced by one of those fanatical anti-abortion groups. It was called *It's Alive* and it was about a murderous baby. The mother had taken an abortion pill to end a pregnancy, but it hadn't had the desired effect. To the contrary, the tiny being had mutated into a monster with the face of a Martian and the teeth of a dog, dead set on killing everything that crossed its path. The second it's born, it kills the doctors and keeps right on killing until it's finally destroyed at the end of the movie. The surprising part is that the mother's character never stops believing throughout the entire movie that the baby can be rehabilitated.

They say that a mother's love is a fail-safe against monsters. Would mine be?

"We're going to be fine," J told me when he came home from his ridiculous telemarketing job. "We'll have a little baby all our own. Won't that be wonderful?"

J had made over eighty phone calls and had sold only three credit cards the entire day. It was a pathetic situation.

That night in bed, while J caressed my flat stomach, I thought of the mothers who killed their children so they wouldn't be taken captive, as had happened, for example, in South Africa. I asked myself to what extremes a mother's love could go. Could you kill children out of love, a misguided love, a genocidal love, but love nonetheless?

In nature, abortion and abandonment of offspring are fairly routine. Among primates, infanticide is common, though the killer tends not to be the mother, but rather a jealous male unrelated to the offspring. Human beings, on the other hand, are the only primates who deliberately kill their children. And women have the advantage over men. We are responsible for the majority of crimes against infants and children.

One of the murderous mothers with the most flair produced by this country where I'd been living for three years, and where I'd probably give birth to my baby, was named Aurora Rodríguez. I'd read about her story for the first time in an article by Rosa Montero published in a popular magazine. Just before the start of the Civil War, the case sent a collective shudder through Spanish society. It came to Aurora Rodríguez that she had a mission: to give birth to a daughter whom she would raise to be a superior woman, capable of saving the world and building a socialist utopia. Aurora thought she was God and to carry out her mission she made use of an accomplice, a man she slept with for the sole purpose of conceiving Hildegart, a prodigy who began receiving instruction when she was still in diapers, who learned to speak five languages by the time she could read and write. By eleven years old she was giving lectures, and at eighteen she had a law degree and was beginning medical school, all under the oppressive inducement of her creator. She joined the Socialist Youth and became a political activist, as well as a scholar in human sexuality. She was a feminist who raised the banner of sexual freedom for women, frequented the intellectual and revolutionary circles of the era and rubbed elbows with H. G. Wells and the celebrated sexologist Havelock Ellis. In all that time, however, Hildegart had not left her mother's home. She and her mother still slept in the same room, and Aurora did not like that her eighteen-year-old daughter was taking the reins of her own destiny and, especially, that she had recently begun wearing a pair of flirtatious earrings that were really quite flattering. Hildegart was in love, she wanted to move out and move on with her life, disregarding the plans her mother had for her. So, early one morning, Aurora shot her several times in the head while she was sleeping. Before being committed for life to a mental institution, the mother declared: "Just like a great artist who can destroy his work if he so chooses because a ray of light reveals an imperfection, that's what I did with my daughter whom I had shaped and who was my work of art." Total madness.

"A little baby all our own." J's words. Yes, I could sense the tremendous power that would be conferred upon me. Giving life had begun to cause me true terror, above all because, for a mother, to give and to take are too close to hand. An absolutely trusting and fragile being depends on your good mood and your better judgment. If you really think about it, it's enough to drive you mad.

The next day, I walked into the metro station and ran into a friend who works for a comic book publisher. As we were waiting for the train, we talked about murderous mothers. The topic was sufficiently pop to fascinate my friend. We talked about Fred and Rose West, the English couple who raped and killed their daughter, along with eight other girls, and continued to live with all of their cadavers until the police dug them up from under the patio of their own home.

"Have you ever heard of Munchausen syndrome by proxy?"

My friend was the type who always brings up some random fact in the middle of a conversation that later turns out to be relevant.

"No . . ."

"I saw it on *House*. The babies are sick but the doctors can't figure out why. They have their suspicions so they set up hidden cameras in the kids' houses and discover that the mothers are harming them."

"What are they doing to them?"

"They starve them, they inject them with urine or feces, they give them medicines that cause fever, vomiting, and diarrhea."

"They inject them with shit?"

"The doctors discovered that the mothers were suffering from Munchausen syndrome by proxy. It's a mental condition that causes them to act with premeditation, to cause the symptoms of an illness in the baby so they can then take it to the emergency room. There are kids who've had dozens of operations before it was discovered that the mother was at fault."

"And what do they get out of it? The mothers, I mean . . ."

"In the hospital, they're the picture of the worried mother. They pretend to be good. They stay by their children's sides. It seems that they like for their children to be suffering from some inexplicable illness, it makes them feel proud. They love the drama of the situation. They're crazy about the attention. Sometimes they'll put their kids on the verge of death in order to save a failing marriage or to gain people's sympathy."

The train arrived at my stop and I said goodbye to my friend.

"Hey," I shouted at him before the doors closed. "I'm pregnant."

In the distance, I could hear him laughing, a demonic laugh like in "Thriller."

We'd done the right thing by having sex at night, because in India they say that during the day the "breath of life" is not present inside the man and, as a consequence, only weak children can be conceived. Another point in our favor was that the highest-quality sperm that a man can produce in his lifetime are obtained when he's about thirty years old. That meant that J had given me the cream of the crop of an entire lifetime.

Of course, if he were carrying it in his belly, everything would be different. You no longer need a uterus, or tubes, or ovaries to carry off a pregnancy. Pretty soon, they'll be able to open up J's belly and implant an egg fertilized in a test tube into the layer of fatty tissue of the peritoneum, just where it surrounds the intestines. Then they'd inject J with a dose of hormones and he'd be both mother and father of our child. Every bit as pregnant and unfeminine as Thomas Beatie, the trans man born with women's genitals who gave birth to a daughter in July 2008.

But for the time being, it's me, the one with the big tits, who's still the mother. Everything had happened inside of me. We were probably still lying there, one of us on top of the other, asking ourselves if it had been good or just okay. Maybe we were talking about the intensity of our orgasms. Or maybe we were already smoking a cigarette or making a sandwich. And inside of me, something was happening: within five minutes, three hundred million sperm had run a marathon and in one hour they were already inside my tubes. Ninety-nine percent of them would die trying, especially the flawed ones, liquidated by my cervical mucus, something like a bouncer at the door of a disco declaring the right to refuse admission. Only a hundred or so had assaulted my delicious ovum, even more selective than my cervix, which in the end allowed just one, the strongest and most intelligent, obviously, to advance with its little tail and plow through with its enormous head filled with information.

And then there was life. From that moment on, everything is written, from the color of its eyes to the timbre of its voice and width of its smile. Soon afterward, the egg was lodged in my uterus and in four weeks it had become an embryo. Those were the microscopic images. And there I was on the outside, enjoying the first month of my adult life without a period, courtesy of my embryo.

Eulalia, the midwife, had weighed me on the first visit. I was starting my pregnancy at 137 pounds. I wasn't exactly skinny. The normal weight gain would be between 20 and 26 pounds. I feared the worst. I had never felt myself so animal. I could detect smells and flavors with renewed intensity, and some that I liked before now sickened me, while others that I disliked before were now glorious.

Read in a hospital booklet: "At two months of pregnancy, the changes you'll be experiencing require just a bit of patience on your part, the slow maturation of this idea: growing a child in body and mind (or soul) requires willingness, disposition, and prudence."

I was sixteen years old and I was in love. We couldn't go to hotels because I looked too young. So we made a bed out of blankets on the cold floor of the landing in a neighboring building. We had brought a box of wine and a couple of joints. It was good enough.

I bled the first time I made love. I don't know why some women bleed and others don't. But I've heard girls proudly report that they didn't bleed. A feminist tactic to diminish the importance of "deflowering"? Did I give too much importance to the vaginal? The truth is, out of distraction more than anything else, I discovered the clitoris fairly late and I spent half my childhood putting things inside my snatch. I'm sorry, but for me, I was moved by that vestige of hymen because, despite my best efforts, I hadn't managed to rupture it myself. He used to paint. Maybe if he hadn't gotten so horribly hooked on drugs he could have become a good illustrator. He liked to draw, and that's why he dipped his finger in my blood and traced the initials of his name on the wall as if signing a painting. A gesture that, despite its backwardness, was almost charming. Many months later, we went on a pilgrimage back to the place where I'd lost my useless virginity to see if his credits were still there. And they were, though somewhat faded. When I told that story about the bloody graffiti to my college friends, they almost murdered me.

We lived very close to the Peruvian Institute for Responsible Parenthood. We started going there because my sex life was just getting started and it seemed to me in poor taste to go to my mother's gynecologist to have my cystitis or recurring yeast infections treated. I don't think I've ever been as irresponsible as I was in those days. I would go to the center, talk to the psychologists and youth counselors, allow myself to be examined by the doctors, try new methods of birth control. They gave me strip upon strip of condoms, but we never used them.

Until it happened. My boyfriend told his mother and she took us to a doctor who had an office on the top floor of a building in San Isidro, a posh neighborhood in Lima. I lay down on the table and they put me to sleep. I didn't feel a thing. I, a very frivolous girl—though not so bad as a girl I knew in college who'd confessed that she'd given her boyfriend a blow job in a doctor's office just like that one, just after having an abortion—asked him to show me what he had taken out of me and the doctor replied curtly that there was nothing to see, that it was just a "ball of blood."

"I still want to see it," I begged.

The doctor stepped to one side and there appeared before my eyes a woman who looked just like Kathy Bates in *Misery*. She was the nurse, holding a bottle that looked like red wine. I was young and in a festive, curious mood. I felt important and I wanted to be fussed over, like when you get your tonsils out. He told me not to eat anything spicy that day, but my mother, who knew nothing about it, served me kebabs with hot chili that night and, since I loved them, I ate them. Nothing happened. I didn't feel a thing. I told my friends about it like just another anecdote from my life: I got my period, I shaved my legs,

I got an abortion. I told them about it because I liked to see their eager faces.

The only thing that remained from that experience was a poem. I titled it "Birth."

Will they wound me
will we wound each other
will I wound you
will I wound myself?

birth, escape

I bring into the light
the night's darkest shadow

I close my eyes
close your eyes too

I know that you, you
exactly you
will not return

my still warm breasts
look strange and absurdly enormous

they split me, Ball of Blood,
like launching you from the water into the great
void
you leave
silhouette
stubborn
Ball of Blood
you leave and I am too alone

The second time I got pregnant wasn't by mistake; we planned it meticulously. At that point, we were seeing each other in secret. My family had forbidden me from seeing him in order to protect me. It was the worst phase of his drug addiction. I was no longer a minor, so I planted myself in front of my parents and told them I was going to have a baby, that he would quit using drugs and we would be happy. My mother told me I had to get an abortion. She explained to me, through tears, that it was for my own good, that I shouldn't be foolish enough to have a baby at my age and "with an addict." But I wasn't interested in being reasonable. I just wanted my love story to continue and a baby could help me achieve that dream. I shut myself in my room, threw myself on the bed, and cried myself to sleep. When I woke up, I heard my father's voice. He was crying too and he was whispering something to me. Surely thinking me still asleep, he was begging me not to have the baby and asking my forgiveness. In the end, I told them I'd do it. I couldn't bear their stricken faces. Although what really decided it for me was a phone call from the baby's father informing me that he was checking into a rehab facility at that very moment, that I should wait for him with our baby, that when he got out, we'd be happy. His intentions were good, but I would have preferred for him to tell me that he had two airplane tickets to Mexico.

My parents took me to another sinister building, this time in the middle-class neighborhood of Jesús María. The doctor was from some NGO and a friend of my parents. Just as they began the curettage, I felt a sharp pain and howled in agony. I was awake. I told the doctor that I couldn't go through with it. The nurse, a total stranger, hugged me out of pure compassion. It would all be over in a few minutes. The suction hurt horribly and I screamed. I thought it was a sign that the baby and I did not want to be parted. The doctor told me: "Don't shout. Abortion is illegal in this country and the neighbors might complain about the noise." I sniffed back my tears in silence, bearing the pain, bearing the disgust and the feeling that, if this wasn't exactly a rape, it sure did feel like one.

I shivered with cold as I left the office. I felt overcome with grief. My parents held me up, took me home, and took care of me as though I had come down with the measles again. I allowed myself to be cared for. There was nothing to do. Mine was a hopeless love. And this had been a second failed attempt.

I promised myself that I would never have another abortion. Two was already a high enough record for my eighteen years. Apparently, I had made use of my rights as an emancipated woman and owner of my own body, although I had the impression that I had done just the opposite.

But four years later I got pregnant again.

And by the boy who had made me forget my first love; in fact, the boy who made me forget what love was altogether. That time, he was the one who took me to get the abortion. Why is there always someone more intelligent than me to drag me off to the slaughterhouse? I guess no one goes to those places cheerfully. A few days before, he had broken my nose with his fist. I had subjected him to long sessions of psychological violence and systematic infidelity. In my worldview, these were ways of avenging his failure or unwillingness to console me with sex when I needed it the most, such as after one of our devastating fights. He hated me and I hated him. Why would we have a child together? We were a disaster. His insistence on the abortion showed excellent leadership on his part, though I applauded it only much later.

Sometimes I wondered if I would be able to have children in the future, if some part of me hadn't been irreparably damaged. Since I don't believe in hell, if it turned out to be the case, it would be—I thought—a punishment tailor-made just for me.

They say that some children carry matricide in their hearts their whole lives. Some act on it and others don't.

I had been reading the Peruvian news on the Internet every morning and I came across this news item: "Giuliana Llamoja Hilares, an eighteen-year-old, savagely murdered her mother on Saturday night after a bitter argument in their house in San Juan de Miraflores. María del Carmen Hilares Martínez (47) died of blood loss after sustaining 65 stab wounds to her body."

Giuliana had been trying on clothes and came downstairs to look at herself in the big living-room mirror. Her mother came in and made a comment about something. Then Giuliana stabbed her 65 times. She said her mother attacked her first.

Back in the era when I lost my virginity, I used a face powder called Angel Face to hide the imperfections of my fifteen-year-old complexion. My mother didn't like it. In truth, the makeup made my skin look fake, but I was convinced I looked good. Teenagers look at themselves in the stepmother's mirror, not the mother's. But she had no reason to understand that; it had been many years since she was a teenager and it irritated her how a girl of my age looks for ways to mitigate her physical insecurities. One afternoon, I sat down at the table and my mother told me that my face looked like a clown's. I didn't see it coming. I ran and locked myself in the bathroom. The tears ran through my mascara. I could have stabbed her in the heart with the butter knife, but instead I threw the compact of face powder out the window of the tenth-floor apartment where we lived.

When we're young, mothers are a terrible hindrance to our plans. Their love is a grenade.

FEBRUARY

I have always lied to my mother. And she to me. How young was I when I learned her language, to call things by other names?

NANCY FRIDAY

"YOU CAN ONLY truly love a mother if you once hated her." I underlined that sentence and closed the book. I had been reading all afternoon in the library, so when I got home, I tried to unwind by putting on one of my favorite movies, *Terms of Endearment*. It didn't work. In that tacky but addictive film, mother and daughter fervently play out the love–hate dynamic. They love each other, but when they're together, it makes for an unmistakably explosive cocktail. That's why they don't live together, although they resort to the telephone almost every day. Every time Debra Winger calls Shirley MacLaine to ask for money or to tell her about the guy she's sleeping with or to announce that she's pregnant for the third time, I understand that that mother–daughter bond has evolved from the umbilical cord to the telephone cord with no significant alteration. Years pass and the two women go on like this, on either end of the phone line, connected by that long, winding, tangled spiral which, to judge by police blotters, has been used dozens of times as a murder weapon or an instrument of suicide. For better or for worse, in every spot on the planet, a mother is making a phone call and a daughter is answering, or vice versa. Although they might both end up hanging up on each other.

It's been eight years since I lived in my mother's house and five since I've lived in the country where my mother lives. I live thousands of miles away from her, and we're separated by an ocean and a twenty-hour airplane flight. We live in different hemispheres. When she's waking up in the morning, I've already had dinner. When I'm going to bed, she's still at the office. I'm outside her field of vision, outside her sphere of influence, and outside her strawberry patch forever.

And yet, sometimes I feel like she's not on the other end of the receiver, but just there in the next room, asking me how everything's going in my life and if I'm eating my vegetables.

Love between two women, especially if one of them gave birth to the other, most resembles passionate love. That's why I was certain that the best thing that could happen to me in life would be to have a son. In my family, men are few and their existence is almost an anomaly. I didn't even have a brother to be able to analyze up close. Women are the most tangible things in my life. And also the most unbearable. That's why, insofar as it was possible, I wanted to spare myself from having to relive the terrifying mother–daughter dialectic, especially from the opposite side.

I love my mother, but she's my mother. I'm supposed to hate her. Like she hated her mother and my grandmother hated my great-grandmother and so on *ad infinitum*. Okay, my mother was not a silent accomplice to the sexual abuse I was subjected to by my father, nor did she stand calmly by while my clitoris was being mutilated so that I could be accepted by the tribe. Nothing like that has happened to me. I don't have, like the majority of people, such serious reasons to hate her. Killing the mother is simply a matter of survival for the human female. I knew very well how to do it (Sylvia Plath *dixit*). I was a professional. I was afraid of turning into my mother but even more afraid that a possible daughter of mine might turn into a daughter like me. Finally, what I feared was the possibility of generating a bad residual copy of myself, capable of hating me even more than I hated myself.

With a boy, with his fat little double chin and his dreamy eyes, all you have to do is teach him how to aim his tiny penis so he doesn't pee on the toilet seat, and he'll love you for the rest of your life. It doesn't matter how bad, ugly, or useless you might be, you've taught him what tits are and now he'll never stop looking for them. We will always be his ideal of a woman, his mommy, his mama, his eternal love, like in that Juan Gabriel song.

In a son, a mother will always have her most loyal defender and in a daughter, her most vicious accuser. I wanted a son whose unconditional love would rescue me from the cliché of the combative relationships between two women.

In just a few weeks, they would tell me what sex organs were developing between my baby's legs. I, an XX, will find out if J's sperm had responded to the challenge with an X or a Y. The little worms marked with a Y are faster, but they're not very hearty and their lives are short. The ones with an X on their foreheads are slower, but they're also stronger and better withstand an acidic environment like that one.

Life depends on the random combination of two letters. The most recent studies contradict the theory that points to the inevitable triumph of the strongest sperm. According to these studies, it is true that only the strongest make it to the ovum, but the one that finally manages to fertilize it is not determined by its own will, but rather by the ovum's, an entity with decision-making powers and clear dislikes, who chooses whom she wants to marry and have children with, softening her cortex to allow him to pass through.

Today, we can determine the sex of our babies with up to eighty percent accuracy. And earlier than ever. There are a series of methods that range from common sense to plain old delirium. Some are based on certain positions in the *Kama Sutra* and a timetable of sexual relations that syncs with ovulation and sounds very strange: if you want a boy, you have to make love one day after ovulation and in a position that allows for deep penetration. If you want a girl, you have to do it four days before ovulation and avoid having an orgasm, limiting yourself exclusively to the missionary position. I doubt there are very many women willing to resign themselves to the missionary position in order to have a boy.

A doctor called "Papa" has also tried to prove that following a certain diet for two and a half months before conception can have good results. For example, according to this guide that quotes Doctor Papa, if you want to have a girl you should eat a lot of dairy products, eggs, fruit and not much meat. And if you want to have a boy, he recommends that you gobble up every kind of meat and sausages you can find.

In case Doctor Papa was on to something, and in clear disregard of the fiber-rich meal plan prescribed by my midwife, I started eating a diet heavy in fat and protein, thinking that I was reinforcing the virility of the boy I hoped I was carrying inside me. Maybe it was just a matter of eating a couple of chorizos in order to fatten up the part that differentiates a boy from a girl. I wondered if, in our transgender world, when thousands of people are transforming or paying to change sexes, it made any sense at all to worry about whether you're having a girl or a boy.

The third month was proving decisive. The guides said it was time to bid farewell to late-night meals, all-nighters, and tobacco. I had already said goodbye to this last without any drama, but now I'd have to discipline myself for all the rest. One of my books noted that "women mature instantaneously, moving from the stage of *young woman* to that of *responsible mother*." As for me, I sometimes felt like a member of that dude's gang in *A Clockwork Orange*, ready to beat a bitch in labor and her still-warm puppies to death with an umbrella. When were the edifying feelings going to arrive?

According to the development curve, the fetus now measured approximately 2.1 inches and weighed two ounces and, I had just learned, not only had nearly complete hands, but also displayed well-defined fingernails. By the end of the third month, the genitals would be fully formed. Maybe the only thing that really mattered was if my descendant, whatever its sex, would bite its nails like I do.

"A woman is her mother," said the poet Anne Sexton with extreme bitterness. I was still feeling a bit disoriented in the mornings, but I think I'd finally managed to overcome the cycle of nausea and overdosing on television. In the days before our trip to Peru, as we were making our final preparations to leave, I had also been devoting a great deal of time to reading books. It was good for me to read in an attempt to understand what was happening to me. I had become a regular at the Francesca Bonnemaison Library, in Barcelona's Borne neighborhood, where their "Dona" section offered a plentiful collection of essays about women and maternity which, through reading and rereading, succeeded in opening new horizons to me. And so, almost by mistake, and thanks to a book of brilliant essays about maternity called *Women and Children First. Essays on Maternity*, I was introduced to the fascinating world of matrophobic literature.

Philosophers, for example, haven't been kind to the figure of the mother. For Rousseau, women, in all cases, are born in order to birth more than four children. For Schopenhauer, women are the snare that perpetuates our species' suffering. According to him, inside every attractive young woman, a mother lies in wait. For Weininger, only two women exist: the mother and the prostitute. But the mother is inferior to the whore because she finds herself dominated by the instincts of her species. A mother should be good, or not be one at all.

Some scholars I read encouraged me not to repress the maternal desire that was taking hold of me and to stop fearing incest, with our small daughter, for example, since they considered it one of the first manifestations of the vital impulse. They drove the point home, denouncing how, in modern Judeo-Christian societies, mothers are conditioned not to love women or women's bodies. Casilda Rodrigáñez's books spoke to me of a "primal maternal sexuality." For her, maternity "should bring about the expansion of eroticism and pleasure, taking pleasure in their babies," and should not remain in the state of "libidinal asepsis" where it is found today.

For some of the feminist intellectuals I read in those days, the legend of The Rape of the Sabine Women—in which Romulus, the first Roman king who, famous for having been nursed by a she-wolf, abducted all the women of a neighboring village in order to populate Rome—was the origin of a maternity hijacked and enforced by men, against which women were rebelling by becoming sterile and having abortions. They praised the Amazons who cut off a breast as an act of protest. Adrianne Rich called for us to rebel against the slavery of our mothers and to liberate ourselves as individuals; to leave behind the victim and the slave we carry inside us, the mother who raised us among sweet little flowers and prejudices, herself a victim of an even more unjust upbringing. Simone de Beauvoir wrote about a mother in one of her novels: " . . . her diffused, indwelling resentment made itself apparent in aggressive forms of behavior—brutal frankness, heavily ironic remarks. With regard to us, she often displayed a cruel unkindness that was more thoughtless than sadistic: her desire was not to cause us unhappiness but to prove her own power to herself."

This distilled venom sounded very familiar to me. We were a community, a network of hate. I, myself, had wanted to negate my mother so I could be a different person, with very little success since, for some time now, I've been stunned to hear that dreaded sentence: "You're just like your mom." A handful of feminists assert that the patriarchy has separated mothers from daughters, but it can't be all the patriarchy's fault. It can't be that simple.

Maternity could also be a subversive political act. Many artists have centered their work on it. *High Tech*, for example, a performance art project by the artist Marta Galán, delves into the representations of maternity through its relationship with technology. It is a "culinary performance" that consists of preparing "tiger's milk" cocktails for the audience, using milk extracted onstage by an electric breast pump. In *My Mother and Me*, the performer Sonia Gómez walks on stage alongside her mother (her actual mother) and makes her listen to Kraftwerk; they dance, pose, fight, converse, bullfight. Sonia undresses in front of her mother, who tells her that she's "too dramatic" and that she should put her clothes back on.

Another great discovery was a short, annotated anthology (edited by Mercedes Bengoechea) of North American female poets that revolved around the painful theme of the mother as "a hole in space": the mother-vampire, the mother-wound, the mother-Medusa, the mother-grave, the mother as a "dark abyss," as a "deep pond" into which the daughter unwittingly plunges. In Sharon Olds's poem, the mother is a sorceress who "can make eggs appear in her hand, pulls silk scarves out of her ear, milk from her nipples," and "can turn anything into nothing."

Someone like the poet Louise Glück could plunge me into despair:

> I don't love my son
> the way I meant to love him.
> I thought I'd be
> the lover of orchids who finds
> red trillium growing
> in the pine shade, and doesn't
> touch it, doesn't need
> to possess it. What I am
> is the scientist,
> who comes to that flower
> with a magnifying glass
> and doesn't leave, though
> the sun burns a brown
> circle of grass around
> the flower. Which is
> more or less the way
> my mother loved me.

Would I be capable of loving my flower without the scalding magnifying glass? If, in fact, every woman IS her mother, then matters were quite clear. If a dirty trick of destiny were to take revenge on me by giving me a girl, I needed to be prepared to drink my own medicine and to give it to my daughter in brimming, bitter strawberry-flavored spoonfuls. I will end up telling her, with brutal frankness and heavily ironic remarks, about the way she laughs, her chewed fingernails, her clown makeup, her inexplicable hairstyles, and she will believe that she was kidnapped by a dictatorship from the arms of her revolutionary mommy and handed over to this fascist stepmother who hates her, before abandoning me forever.

No, it wasn't hatred, it was fear, just fear of being a pale reflection. That's why daughters have to do everything inside out, the opposite way that our mothers would have wanted. I was running the risk of becoming one of them. Please, gods, storks, do not send me a daughter.

Send me a healthy, hairy boy.

The morning of my first ultrasound, I woke up especially hungry. I chewed on a cracker to quell the discordant void I felt in my stomach when I woke up. I bathed and looked at myself naked, in profile, in the mirror. I confirmed that it was still there. In the past few days, I had finally noticed a hint of a belly that began high in my abdominal area, separating it in two. It didn't look like a beer belly, or a pregnant belly either, strictly speaking, but there it was, seeking its place. Overall, I was still me, my body covered in drops of water that reflected my solitary reflection dozens of times in the mirror. True, I had listened to the sound of another heartbeat alongside my own, but in order to close this vicious circle of incredulity, I had to first see that face, just as I was looking at myself right now. That's why it was such an important day.

I wouldn't be going to Eulalia's office as I usually did. I was supposed to take a little tour of the hospital where, according to plan, my baby would be born.

Maternity is not just a concept to philosophize over and a theme for poems and self-help books or performance art; it's also a three-story building very close to Camp Nou. There, they would take down my medical history and perform my first-trimester ultrasound.

Barcelona Maternity was a good place to give birth. It wasn't at all like the hospitals that we called maternity wards in South America, places that were basically charities where low-income women and teen mothers went to give birth. No, this was one of those public hospitals with all the guarantees and the luxury of being one of the few in Catalonia with its own natural birth protocol. That sounds complicated but really it only means that, if I felt like it, I could give birth there without anesthesia, like a woman out in the middle of a field.

I'd heard about natural birth, but when I learned that I'd be having my baby at Barcelona Maternity, I truly paid attention to it for the first time. Apparently, natural birth didn't only mean a vaginal birth, it also represented the most avant-garde among pregnant women, neo-hippies or otherwise, who believed in an alternative birth, far from the cold hospital dynamic that tends to surround labor and delivery and sees the birthing mother as a patient or just another sick lady to stick tubes in. The theory suggested that it is possible to give birth without anesthesia and without pain and that you could actually even have orgasms during the birth. A lot of young women these days are choosing to have births that follow the normal physiological process, without medical intervention, only making use of hospital support in the case of emergency. Giving birth at home, like our grandmothers did, or in water, was even more natural, but also more risky, and so more and more people were deciding to give birth at Barcelona Maternity. It offered rooms specially equipped for giving birth, with a bed you could squat on, a tub with hot water, an enormous ball you could bounce around on to help with the expulsion process, and mirrors that allowed you front-row seats to see the crowning moment. You would not be attended to by a gynecologist, but rather by an intuitive and experienced midwife like in the old days. With this kind of birth, termed "respectful birth," and in contrast to the medicalization of "the experience of giving birth to a life," the pregnant woman is not subjected to the medical-hygienic practices that are traditionally considered obligatory for a birth; that is, she is not shaved or given a questionable enema, much less an episiotomy, which is an incision in the perineum.

If there was one thing in the world that I truly feared—more than the idea that a being from another dimension might come out of there, more than the thought of motherhood itself, more than earthquakes and airplanes—it was an episiotomy. The manuals sold it as nothing more than an insignificant little cut between the vagina and the anus that would enlarge the opening of the birth canal through which your baby's giant head was supposed to appear, thus preventing possible tearing. But in reading about natural birth, I came across some very disturbing information: not only were episiotomies painful—in the haste of birth, nurses made savage cuts and repairs that were slow to heal, causing women discomfort that could last for weeks or months, leaving them unable to sit down, hampering their ability to care for and nurse their babies—they were harmful and unnecessary. Apparently, they were still done solely per protocol and to speed up the birth process, even when the situation did not require it. And it was a fact that they weren't necessary in more than 90 percent of births. Even a tear and a few stitches were preferable.

For some women, an episiotomy has changed their lives forever. They are victims of profound physical damage and psychological trauma. I don't want to go into too much detail, but there are women for whom it takes months before they can make love again, others whose vaginas ended up asymmetrical, disfigured, and one poor woman whose vagina and anus became one and the same. The horror, the horror . . .

I decided that I should try for a natural birth, or at the very least, avoid that slash at all costs.

At the video store on the corner by my house (which is so freaky it has a section just for Tom Berenger films) there is also a section specializing in dramas about lost children, kidnapped children, disappeared children, adopted children, etc. It's a very popular genre. I imagine that losing a child, or rather having a child taken from you, is one of the most powerfully entrenched fears in the collective unconscious and fertile ground for all sorts of morbid

fictions. In Polanski's film *Rosemary's Baby*, the Devil himself and a satanic sect comprised of the protagonist's own
husband and their neighbors want to take her baby away
from her. The protagonist lives permanently anesthetized
and, at the end, they succeed in taking her baby away.
The most horrifying thing in the film isn't whether or
not the baby is the Devil's spawn, but rather the appearance of some nasty types—call them Satan, an asshole
husband, society, the government, the Church, doctors,
your mother-in-law, your neighbors, Tom Cruise—who
want to play the role of mother for you. In Tarantino's
Kill Bill, there's another mother whose child is stolen, but
unlike the fragile and drugged Rosemary, Beatrix Kiddo,
thirsting for blood and revenge, embarks on a brave and
monumental quest to get him back. I wondered how many
times the Devil would tempt me and how many times I'd
be capable of killing for my little cub. I was going to need
to learn some martial arts.

J took the day off to come with me to the first sighting of
our baby, so there we both were waiting our turn, surrounded by other aspiring parents. To tell the truth, the
majority of them were in much more cumbersome situations than I was. Next to me was a legion of big-bellied
women having serious trouble breathing, moving, and

basically doing things that before were simple and now looked like monumental challenges.

"How many months are you?"

The woman who'd spoken was positively overflowing, her cheeks were round, her legs, arms, and feet almost elephantine and, in addition to supporting an eight-month belly, she had two little girls clinging to her neck.

J narrowed his eyes at me. Just then, I heard them calling my name. For a few seconds, I thought that the voice was coming from my belly. I stood up like a soldier at attention and followed the white-clad lady to the exam room. She gave me a robe and asked me to take off my underwear. I must have looked at her strangely because she went on:

"You're in the first trimester, right?"

"Yes."

"At this stage, the ultrasound is transvaginal."

Of course. Not even now, with my small inhabitant, was I going to be free of the devices. The next ultrasound would be through the abdomen but, for now, I needed to shuck my thong and stretch out next to the ultrasound machine. The sonographer, who is not a doctor or a mid-wife or a nurse and God only knows what she actually is, but anyway, she put the device inside me while J and I locked eyes on the small and beat-up looking black and white screen in front of us. For an instant, while she moved her wand around inside me looking for signs of life, I thought, it's just like the time when it took Eulalia a while to find those elusive heartbeats, that she was going to say that there was nothing there, it's a mistake, I'm sorry, Ma'am, you're as hollow as a coconut.

Electra killed her mother, Clytemnestra, to avenge her father, Agamemnon. So much for Greek tragedy.

Agrippina was mother to a son and she wasn't exactly a happy woman. Her son's name was Nero, a fat little pyromaniac and Roman emperor. Agrippina wanted to be Empress while still being a mother and she ended up not only committing incest with her son, but also being killed by him. Another kind of eternal love. So much for history.

Athena was born from the head of Zeus and is, therefore, a goddess without a mother. The goddess of wisdom. So much for mythology.

Selma from the Lars von Trier film *Dancer in the Dark* dies on the gallows for trying to get some glasses for her son. So much for movies.

And what kind of mother would I be?

Although you still can't see it on the ultrasound, my fetus is already biologically a man or woman in the making.

Unless the future baby is a hermaphrodite, like a snail or a lizard, but the probability is very low. Since I still had to wait eight more weeks to find out my baby's sex, I tried to calm myself and trust in nature's expertise and the vindictive power of myth, movies, and universal history.

Then, live and direct, a news channel exclusive, without commercial interruptions, by means of a somewhat fuzzy transmission, from a place not unlike a remote constellation, in the middle of the black nothingness of my insides, it appeared. There it was, minute but visible, like a pea on a plate, bound to my flesh like a Siamese twin, throbbing and twitching on its bedroll at the slightest tremor caused by us from the outside. It was moving but I couldn't feel it yet. J and I looked at each other, wordless. If I was a galaxy, it was my solitary inhabitant, unaware that we were spying on it in this intrauterine *Truman Show* through a camera hidden in my vagina.

It was true. I was pregnant, as real as it was irreversible. It was almost certain that it wasn't going anywhere, not unless I wanted it to. It would dedicate itself to growing and growing until it came out of its hiding place and took over my entire life.

"Is this it?" said J to be certain, pointing excitedly at a white dot on the screen.

The professional merely nodded. She was very busy dictating strange terms to her assistant. I adjusted my glasses and looked at the white spot. Finally, she spoke:

"Single fetus with active heartbeat, appropriate size, moving spontaneously and approximately twelve and a half weeks gestation," she dictated. "We'll give you a report with the results."

"Is everything okay?"

"Everything is okay, Ma'am."

As a souvenir, she gave us what would be considered the first photograph of my child. Not a fantasy seahorse: at least in the photo, it was a rock obstructing the mouth of a vortex. I put it in my pocket and spent the rest of the afternoon looking at it while I was packing to get on the airplane that would take me to Lima.

J took me to a seamstress. It was odd because I didn't remember having anything that needed mending. The seamstress's house was on a small street, a sort of dead-end alleyway. She was inside, an older woman, her hair completely white, sitting in a wheelchair with a colorful patchwork quilt over her legs. Her home was modest and there was nothing but a big table and old clothes everywhere. I asked J why he had brought me there and he asked me to just wait. The woman stood up and went over to a cabinet in the back of the room. She came back with a spool of flesh-colored thread and with several needles in her mouth. She took one out and held it up. "It's a diamond-tipped needle," she said to J. He nodded. The old woman asked me to please remove my underwear and lie down on the table. I did. Then she began to sew my vagina with short, tight stitches, until it was completely sewn shut in a long, black seam. She cut the thread with her teeth.

I woke up. I was still on the airplane.

Lima, my mother, were only two hours away.

4

MARCH

WAKING UP IN YOUR childhood bed next to your husband is a strange way of coming full circle or biting your own tail. Sleeping here has been like sleeping in a sort of sanctuary, something halfway between the museums of natural history and archaeology. The museum of my childhood illuminated by the amber glass of my windowpane: posters, letters returned to their anxious sender, dolls. A collection of pieces with the little "do not touch" sign attached.

It wasn't the first time I'd slept with a man in that bed, although it was the first time I'd done so with a man I called my husband. In fact, during one period of time, which I think of as the apex of my life as a spoiled daughter, my mother used to bring breakfast in bed to me and the boy I'd brought home the night before. It wasn't exactly that she was a liberal mother. It had been hard for her to accept that I was sexually active, but we all know that there's nothing better for a mother than to have you home under her own roof, even if what you do under that roof is, for example, anal sex.

The reeducation of a mother is slow, but it does bear fruit.

Being here didn't feel at all transgressive, but it did feel nostalgic. I've always been turned on by sexual situations in domestic spheres. My models were the North American girls from the 50s who let themselves be felt up in front of the TV, who took out their gum before kissing and stuck it underneath the coffee table, who unbuttoned their blouses to reveal their gigantic brassieres. That's why, for me, being in my parents' house now had a twisted, unmentionable plus side. My dog barking, my mother's distant voice, the clanging of the plates in the dishwasher were like an aphrodisiac music. It must be that they immediately connected me to times of greater spiritual arousal, the happy days when I rolled about on the sofa while my grandmother watched soap operas and I had to keep my ears pricked for the sound of her slippers shuffling toward me.

In some way, pre-penetration sexuality under conditions of maximum alert is like a lost El Dorado for some women and, during the preamble to every sexual encounter, we tend to reactivate the guilty desire and delicious paranoia of our patrolled pubescence inside the forbidden realm of the family home. To be on the verge of being discovered unleashed in me, years later, a massive wave of estrogen, greater than that in a cow drugged with Yohimbine. I turned over and came up against J's supine, sweaty body. For a moment, he took his warm hands from between my legs and stroked them across my face, moving my long hair to one side so he could kiss me.

In the past two months, sex had become a sporadic and scheduled activity. The nausea killed my desire and desire made me nauseated. When we did make love, we always ended up talking about the baby, things like:

"Am I hurting you?"

"No, but I think you're crushing its skull."

And we'd leave off at that. We were careful not to inconvenience it with any strange positions. Also, although it was still too early to feel its presence between us, we also couldn't act like it didn't exist. Waking up in my childhood bedroom that morning was the first time in many days that we felt a true hunger and desire to go all the way.

J got on top of me without much preamble. My old bed started to creak. Finally, another monster inside of me had awoken. In invisible combat with the new creature, it had won or else they had fused into a single, desirous beast. The last thing I heard was my mother's voice calling us to breakfast and my dog howling.

I was back.

My friends Irene and Violeta were waiting for me with their boys at La Marina Lighthouse in Miraflores to spend a sunny afternoon in the park. Violeta's son would have been about six months old and he was stretched out on his stomach on the grass, playing with a ball. Irene's son had just turned one and he was walking around carrying a stick. They were both friends from my college days and it had been a few years since I'd seen them. Though I had followed the saga of their pregnancies, and then the day-to-day of their babies' lives, through emails and photos, it was the first time I would get to see them in person in their new role as mothers. From the first days of my pregnancy, they had been my main advisors.

Brief biographies of my two friends:

Irene, small, with round eyes, is a painter and lives with her husband and son abroad, in a small city in the South of France.

Violeta, lanky, with Asian features, is a linguist, lives in Peru in the middle-class neighborhood of Jesús María, and is a single mother.

That's just for a start.

Irene, who had chosen to stop working in order to dedicate herself body and soul to being a mother and homemaker, was a fervent defender of natural birth and an active member of La Leche League, an international organization that brings together women who share a militant passion for breastfeeding and supports various programs to promote it. Thanks to The League, Irene had been able to get through the loneliness of living far away from her family in a foreign country but, above all, it had given her a way to share her logical doubts and fears as a first-time mother. In finding other women dedicated to their children, she also began to free herself of the first-world stigma of being a woman who "doesn't work." To my mind, the existence of this kind of association was almost as rare as discovering a Roller Coaster Enthusiasts Club or a Banana Lovers Guild. I was almost as surprised to learn that, every Thursday, Irene got together with other women from her neighborhood to talk about their boobs and their milk.

I can say honestly that the fact of Violeta's motherhood was partially because of me. It happened a few years back. In those days, I was working as an editor, writing bizarre news stories for a newspaper in Lima. That night, I was working on a particularly sensationalistic one, the title of which was going to be something like: "How Women

Score in Lima" (I've never been very imaginative when it comes to themes), and it consisted of going with a group of girlfriends to a series of bars known as hook-up spots and then writing about the experience in great detail. During our bar tour, Violeta zeroed in on a tall, well-built stud of a man, whom she went to bed with that very night, much to the delight of my long-suffering pen, and with whom she fell deeply in love, throwing overboard her unhappy, sexless marriage. From this reasonable yet futureless adultery was born the beautiful little boy who was now sitting on the grass like a tiny Buddha.

Irene and Violeta had put up with all my questions and had been good friends in sharing their infinite wisdom with me. That day would be no exception. We talked about our pregnant-woman obsessions.

"Ooof, I don't know, Wiener . . . "

Violeta is an intellectual but she's used to dealing with the common folk, so her humor is a mixture of incisive wit and vulgarity. Irene likes to live in accordance with her principles and, while that's still a distant paradigm for me, I have to admit that it's a value on the rise. Violeta began with her little *boutades*:

"Okay, obsession number one: kill the baby's father. Obsession number two: kill my mother. Obsession number three: have sex."

"Yesterday, I had sex with J for the first time in weeks . . . " I confessed to them.

"Yum."

"We almost never have sex. It never even occurs to us. Especially after the birth. I had to enroll in tango classes."

"Tango classes. . . . Why?"

"So I wouldn't forget how to move my ass," said Irene. "I would have cheated on him in a heartbeat except it's not as easy to fuck a random stranger there as it is here."

" . . . I had a couple of second acts with a few old lovers during the first four months. Then, zero activity," said Violeta. "None. Zilch. I haven't had sex in almost a year . . . "

"A year?! Don't fuck with me . . . "

"I hate that I'm already not having sex at my age."

"It has to be temporary . . . "

"Sometimes I masturbate just so I don't forget how, but I have to admit that most of the time, I just fall asleep in the middle of it."

We laughed, looking at the boys, who had started to interact with one another.

"Hey, if you count the nine months, plus the thirteen months since he was born . . . "

"That's almost two years! You poor thing . . . "

"You guys are scaring me, seriously . . . "

After sex, we veered into the swampy territory of our bodies. It was the first time that I didn't feel like I had to make excuses to my friends about my current physical condition: it went beyond me and what I wanted for myself. In fact, it was the first time that I didn't feel paunchy. A contradiction, given the curved belly I was sporting. But there you have it. I'd never had a Santa Claus belly, just a somewhat pudgy stomach, a family trait. But I'd always felt chubby. And now I wasn't a chubby chick. Now I was a pregnant chick. My real gut was now hidden behind my virtual gut.

"I'm scared that no one will be able to love me with this stomach."

Violeta said this and suddenly lifted her T-shirt and showed us the ravaged surface of her abdomen. It seemed incredible that my friend's belly had once been a flat plain of taut skin with a sweet little bikini-ready bellybutton. Her stomach had stretched so much that, toward the eighth or ninth month, the skin had torn. The skin on her stomach had run like a pair of pantyhose. It was as striped as a tiger, or worse, it looked like a pair of tigers had gotten into a brawl on her belly.

"Sometimes I think that someone will fall in love with my unique features," Violeta went on, thoughtfully. "If my son loves them so much, someone else will discover the virtues of my new geography. In fact, one of these days, I'm going to do fifteen sit-ups . . . "

The sun was about to dissolve into the ocean, and we decided we should get up and move around a bit. To break the reigning sense of melancholy, we walked toward a shopping center and scarfed down gigantic ice cream sundaes with whipped cream and fudge.

That night, J told me that he would love me with stretch marks, with warts, with varicose veins, and with pimples. That same night, I started to rub snail extract cream onto my belly. On TV they said it would work.

The "maternal-fetal bond" I'd heard so much about was at work inside me. In a strange way, I was experiencing a sort of fetal regression, a return to the womb, to my mother's house, to the country of my youth, to my horrible city. Lima was a fucking time tunnel. Lima was a pretty psychoanalyst, with short hair, small tits, who had studied at the Universidad Católica (my university), who had sat next to my couch and hypnotized me with her perfume in order to wrest truths from my tongue.

I had returned to a city in which Adriana no longer existed. She had left through a window. It wasn't our first casualty in that metropolis of suicides, either. There is a bridge here that the most desperate used to throw themselves off of. One day, the authorities got tired of scraping guts off the pavement and ordered huge glass walls to be erected around the bridge. A cruel architecture. Since the walls are made of glass, you can still see the void, but now you can no longer embrace it. I went to the cemetery to read a poem I had written to Adriana. Pregnant women also go to the cemetery and vomit on the gravel. It was a poem in which I remembered a night in Usquil, a small village in the northern mountains of Peru, near where the poet César Vallejo had been born. It was the Friday of Easter Week. I had been watching *Ben-Hur* in a movie theater that was a stone house with a television in it. When I came out, I ran into Adriana and the others, sitting in circles on the grass. They had found fireflies and some of them were in her hair like phosphorescent ribbons. One had landed on her nose and it glowed there like a spot of glitter. She was laughing, she looked beautiful, resplendent. We talked about bioluminescence. Someone said that it was the phenomenon that made the fireflies glow, and that they used it to attract males. A question of chemistry. That was all. We were all smoking, so it seemed to more than one of us that we were in a movie. Everyone was happy, except me. I always think I'm the only one who isn't happy, but just now I think that maybe it isn't so true. That's what my poem's about. About being a voyeur of happiness.

I asked Adriana how she had made me believe that she was floating when in reality she was trembling. And she answered that at first it was a game and in the end it was a trick. I used to think that behind these bars there was a garden where everyone was having fun except me. And Adriana was having fun too. That's why I asked her. The trick was called lithium and carbamazepine. One day, when I was already in Spain, the guy who was her ex-boyfriend by then called me to let me know that Adriana had been admitted to a psychiatric hospital, like a firefly inside a box. There, during that era of electroshock and jailers, she wrote about her hospital bed, a bed alongside other, identical beds, filled with other, identical people, to which she did not want to return.

One morning, she went out for a walk through Miraflores, something she did to ward off depression, but that time it didn't work. She walked into a mediocre hotel called Sol y Luna, on gray Angamos Avenue, rented room 406, and fifteen minutes later threw herself into the void. An unremarkable police blotter sidenote.

Four months later, a pregnant lady in a cemetery was trying to see or not to see the world from that window, reading out loud one of the hundreds of poems that Adriana never published:

> And in the windows
> the men observe the city
> [. . .]
> and they do not suspect
> that above them
> the rooftops
> are
> the dance floors.

How funny our youth is, how stupid. Too many neon lights, not enough fireflies.

Little by little, the cloud of death seemed to be dissipating from the dirty white sheet that is the sky in Lima, a veritable shroud. My father had beaten colon cancer a few weeks earlier and I was seeing the results with my own eyes. They hadn't even had to give him chemo. He still read five newspapers every morning, working during the day and playing solitaire on the computer between writing articles. I, who had become a journalist to be like him, had not lived through his illness up close. When you're far away, you miss out on the good and the bad things that happen to the people you love. That had been a relief, by which I mean that it had been a relief not to see him suffer, grow thin, be afraid; but I would have liked to be there when he needed me most. Instead, I'd been on the other side of the ocean, bedridden after my operation, pregnant and unemployed, and hearing about his progress remotely over the telephone.

The day I married J, fifteen days before I left, alone, for Barcelona, my Dad wrote me a letter. It said: "Up the steps to the airplane goes my eldest daughter, who will always be my little girl. Little by little she's been leaving me and I have watched her go, helpless. She's leaving, the one who made me a father, the purest thing I've been in my life. She is leaving and my heart will feel her absence. Now I will have to talk to her through my thoughts and wait in silence, as I alone know how to do."

I sat on his lap, his legs still strong, and I pecked his mole as I've done since I was a child. My father's mole makes a magical sound. Well, the truth is that I peck and he whistles and I pretend I don't realize it.

In a few months, someone will arrive who will make me a mother.

And I won't be a little girl anymore.

I don't want to be a grown-up.

I don't ever want to lose him.

Ever since I'd arrived, my mother had been spoiling me, making my favorite dishes, fussing over me and my symptoms. As always, I responded to her demonstrations of love with the cruel sarcasm of a latter-day rebel. I don't know what went on between us that, together, we unleashed some strange energy. Maybe we were competing to see who could make the other submit. I resisted setting aside the squabbles of my adolescence and embarking on a more mature relationship with her. She continued to see me as the fifteen-year-old who wore face powder that made her look like Michael Jackson.

Every morning, I stood in front of the mirror to see how the outfit I'd chosen for the day looked on me. Suddenly, my mother came out of the kitchen, saw me and shot off:

"What are you doing with that skirt over your pants? It looks hideous."

She said it in such a familiar way that it paralyzed me, but I still managed to answer her. I had left her strawberry patch forever many years ago, but she didn't appear to have noticed. I looked her up and down, pausing for a long time on her striped blouse and extra-large pants.

"Have you looked at yourself in the mirror, Mom?"

She lowered her gaze for the first time since my return, for the first time since we'd started this game that had lasted my entire life.

I had wounded her.

I was about to embark on my triumphal retreat, but I noticed that she was crying. I no longer felt so triumphant.

"Please don't cry."

"What did I do wrong? Why did you turn out like this? Shit just flows from your mouth."

This was the opportunity we'd been awaiting for so long. She would vent, tell me how complicated it is being a mother, just as hard, or even harder, than being a daughter. She would justify her harassment by telling me how hostile my grandmother had been with her. We would embrace and beg each other's forgiveness.

We had both inherited a tendency for destructive criticism from my grandmother. Both of us, like her, could be very sweet, but when our tempers got the better of us we were direct, savage, and degrading.

During my visit to Lima, not much was left of my grandmother, who had been severe with her own children and indulgent with her grandchildren, who had laughed at our mischief and offered us her ample lap and her cooking. Now she lay in her bed, in a wallpapered room patterned with a spring landscape filled with yellow flowers, not able to speak or move after several strokes, cared for by my grandfather and two nurses. She would die soon after.

My mother once confessed to me that her mother found fault with her in almost everything; one day she told her that if she kept coming home late, "like a man," the neighbors were going to think she was a slut.

Even though she grew up hearing this kind of thing, my mother kept coming home late and staying out at gatherings with the other young people she called "comrades." She dreamed of bringing about the continental revolution that would end injustice, although afterward she would have to go home and sleep in her poor, Catholic girl's bed. It didn't scare her that her mother or her neighbors might think she was a slut. It also didn't scare me that my mother considered me a producer of verbal shit.

Without looking away, I grabbed my purse and held it across my belly. I thought I would walk out the door without saying a word, but I couldn't.

I went over and gave her a kiss. She stood quietly in front of the mirror.

Brief inventory of my previous experiences related to motherhood: 1) A bunny when I was three: attachment, powerful feelings of tenderness and fascination; sudden disappearance of the bunny, my parents explain to me that he had to go because his mommy missed him very much, I realize that I am not his mommy: disappointment, but I understand the (false) situation rationally and I forget quickly. 2) A dog when I was fifteen: cocker spaniel, caramel colored, nervous and epileptic; a boy I'm dating tells me he thinks my dog is homosexual and I can verify that it's true; one day, we take him to the vet for a bath and he never comes back; he dies because of the vet's negligence, he'd drugged him in order to bathe him (that son of a bitch) and he overdid it. 3) Another dog when I was twenty: also a cocker spaniel, caramel colored, given to us by the son of a bitch veterinarian; the dog has major behavioral disorders, he's incapable of obeying and no one can teach him anything, he shits on the dining-room table, pees on my bed, once almost rips my ear off, they rush me to the emergency room, they sew up my earlobe with five stitches: to this day my earrings are perpetually asymmetrical. 4) A cat when I was twenty-five: a mongrel, I buy him in the market for ten *soles* out of jealousy because the alley cat that visits us and to whom I've grown attached one day decides to go with my neighbor, apparently because she feeds him better-quality food; he lives with me and J for two years; we decide to travel to Spain and don't know what to do with him; disappearance of the cat, no one explains anything to me, there are no made-up tales, I think he abandoned us before we could abandon him, J thinks he's in cat heaven. 5) A plant when I was thirty: I buy it from a gypsy woman at the entrance of the Encantes market; I don't even know what kind of plant it is, it's green, obviously; as it grows I notice that it's a climbing plant, it almost dies several times, it clearly needs to be repotted but I never have the time or the money to do it, I water it every once in a while; one day I move and leave it behind, a friend moves into my old house, tells me that she's transplanted it, I go to visit my friend and I see my plant, it has flowers, it is no longer my plant.

My résumé as a guardian of living beings wasn't much to be proud of. With inanimate objects, the situation was different, though I don't know if for the better. My dolls, teddy bears, stuffed ducks, Barbies, and other little play-things were my true school of horrors. In this particular *Toy Story*, I subjected my Barbies to long sexual sessions with castrated Kens or I made them star in plots full of natural disasters. I stripped the clothes off Allan, one of my baby dolls, and then dismembered and ultimately decapitated him like Túpac Amaru with a pacifier. His body parts were always strewn about different parts of my room and they never came back together. When I became a teenager, I committed incest with one of my children: my Bomboncito Farmer Boy, a doll as big as a three-year-old with red hair made of yarn that I used as a partner to

masturbate with. What would Bomboncito say to the tin
soldier and the rest of his siblings at the end of the day,
when they came back to life to tell of their adventures
with the girl who was now asleep in her bedroom?

I hope he spoke well of me. If not, he'd be a total
hypocrite.

Lima was also that place that a poet given to mischief
called "the city where there is no love." I noted that the
majority of my friends were no longer there: my gang
from the university was scattered all over the world, full
of voluntary casualties, as I've said, and the ones who
remained were just contacts in my inbox: so close but yet
so far. I didn't even have a million friends on Facebook I
could brag to about being a good person. My youth, which
I'd left behind just three years ago in this very place, had
been swallowed up by the earth. Some friends had trave-
led, others had died, there were a few who didn't want to
see me and a few I didn't want to see. My girlfriends who
didn't have kids were doing yoga or meditation. A few couples had somehow managed to stay together and others
were now nothing but ashes. None of my gay friends had
come out of the closet and the straight ones still hadn't
resigned from *El Comercio*, the newspaper we worked for
once upon a time. None of my ex-boyfriends upon whom

I believed I'd made a lifelong impression tried to contact me. And my lovers even less. No one interrupted their routine to spend time with me, not even my own family. Except for two friends who also lived in Barcelona (and with whom I'd met up in Lima to take our revenge on the privations of Barcelona in one of their beach houses), people were only available at night, on schedules that were not suitable for pregnant ladies. I thought I'd be able to party like before but, if I didn't fall asleep first, my vague attempts to go out for drinks always ended in a kind of dietary lack of restraint that I tried to satiate with sandwiches overflowing with sauce. My belly started to expand. Instead of fighting against it, as I had done all these years, I began to embrace it. I devoured every kind of Peruvian food I came across and almost upchucked my little tenant after eating a plate of ceviche with black clams in the market in my old neighborhood. I devoted myself to eating and indulging my cravings. One day, I would want a caramel apple in the park, another day a meat empanada and passion fruit juice in the Plaza de Armas; I'd be tempted by a breakfast of *chicharrones* in the Callao district and two cherimoyas as dessert in the dining room of my house. A hamburger with bacon on the corner of my alma mater, barbecued chicken with chili at the shopping center near Asia Beach, a *manjar blanco* ice cream in an ice cream shop that no longer exists. It occurred to me that Peru's explosive gastronomy would be the death of my baby one of these days.

Although it was difficult, I threw a baby shower at which I tried to disguise the lack of real friends by inviting legions of my sister's friends and my cousins' girlfriends. Everyone insisted that I should have one of those gatherings meant to rake in the largest possible quantity of baby products. You should take advantage of being in Lima, they said, it will be hard for people to send you things from here when the time comes. I remembered that there was no similar tradition in Barcelona, so it seemed like a good idea to me despite some measure of secret shame. I sent an online invitation that I'd made myself, a sort of collage with a photo of J and one of me from when we were children. A text bubble came out of my mouth like in the comics: "I'm pregnant!" my child-self shouted into the incredulous face of the chubby-legged little J. On the day, I opened all kinds of gifts. A baby shower is a lot like a bridal shower, except instead of smiling penises and red thongs, what emerge from the gift wrapping are strange artifacts like nasal aspirators or a little chest in which to keep the stub of the umbilical cord. Instead of steamy scenes, there are drooly ones and, instead of moans, there are tender oohs and ahhs at the sight of a little bear bib.

The stripper is definitely you yourself, as you bare that part of your soul that should always remain clothed.

Mine was a fairly premature baby shower. Generally speaking, they're done in the sixth or seventh month, when the baby's sex is already known. Forewarned, my guests bestowed upon me baby clothes in "unisex" colors such as white, yellow and green. Only one of my aunts wagered it would be a girl and dared to gift me a pink onesie with little flowers on it. The afternoon progressed amid canapés and non-alcoholic drinks. That night, I did an inventory of my acquisitions. With alarm, I realized that the baby things completely filled the largest suitcase we'd brought. It had more clothes than I did, and it didn't even exist.

In the first image I have of my mother, she's aiming a gun at me. It's not a metaphorical image but a real one. She's about ten in the black-and-white photo and my grandfather is helping her hold up the gun and she's looking off into some point in the distance and the gun is aimed straight at the camera. My old photo album begins with that photo. I don't know why it's in there. I think I stole it from my grandfather's photo album. I liked the irony of that image: a little girl in her Sunday best learning how to shoot a gun with her father. A girl who would become my mother. In the next photo in the album, there's the same girl, with almost the same sweet expression, nursing a baby. A baby that was me. They took that photo of my mother in the hospital, the day after she gave birth. My mom looks tired but happy, like in diaper ads. While I nurse intently, my tiny, dark hand clutching her breast, just a small, black head squeezed between a teat and the world, she's looking at my father, his hair in a 70s style, and she's saying something to him.

In another photo, I had transformed into a flower with pink petals and a red stem for a school play. I remember that my mother had made me that costume and, since she hadn't been able to find the regulation green tights, she had lovingly made me a pair of green crepe paper pants that ripped the first time I bent over, thus revealing my red underpants. I was very embarrassed, but what kid dressed as a flower isn't? I finally found the photo I was looking for: the one of the field trip to Chosica in first grade, the photograph of humiliation. In the background are my classmates, including my best friend, enjoying a swim in the pool and laughing raucously; in the foreground: me, fully dressed, with two pigtails and the saddest face I've ever seen in my entire life, hugging the bronze statue of the little angel who's watering the pool with his penis. I had a cold. I remember that my parents had generously agreed to let me go on the field trip but they didn't want me to swim in the pool for fear I'd get worse.

I decided several things about my future that day: I would never make a costume for my child, I would never send him on a field trip with a cold, and I would teach him how to shoot.

The symbolic return to my mother's house grew intense when a slight pain in my back that I'd had since Barcelona turned debilitating due to inflammation of my sciatic nerve. Sciatica is fairly common among women entering the third trimester and up to thirty percent of pregnant women suffer from it. It's a pain that begins in your butt and radiates down your leg. Apparently, the muscles in my back had contracted because of the sudden excess weight, and my sedentariness had only made the problem worse. My fetus was putting pressure on the nerve and I was being torn apart. Added to this was the intense pain in the so-called "pelvic floor," that is, the pubis and the vagina, due to the twisting of the ligaments. In other words, my pelvis was expanding thanks to a hormone called "relaxin," in order to prepare the way for that big head. The average space between the bones of a non-pregnant woman is between 4 and 5 millimeters and, during pregnancy, it's normal for that space to expand by

2 to 3 millimeters. An insignificant figure that nevertheless made me go berserk.

It came as no surprise to me that my mother would take
over responsibility for the lame daughter who must once
again depend on others after years of self-management
abroad. The first thing she did was to take me to her most
trusted doctor's office: The Peruvian-Japanese Polyclinic.
After a decade of *fujimorismo*, certain habits had become
very deeply entrenched. The main one in this situation
was that the clinic wasn't expensive and they offered
physical therapy. So there I was, at the climax of my vaca-
tion, waiting my turn and talking to my mother in a room
filled with people who used orthopedic products.

"You were born with jaundice. Your entire body was
orange and they took you away from me and I didn't see
you until the next day."

Jaundice causes an abnormal yellow color due to an
excess of bilirubin in the blood that a newborn's liver is
unable to process. It's treated with phototherapy (exposure
to light) and, in its mildest form, it lasts only a few days.
Almost all babies have it, and my baby probably would too.

"I didn't know what I felt when I saw you."

"You didn't feel love right away?"

"No. I just wanted nothing bad to happen to you and
I waited for you so I could hug you and protect you."

"Sort of an animal reaction . . . "

"Yes, like an animal with its young. I'm sure that night you spent without me you missed me and that's where the poet was born."

My mother has always believed that I'm a poet. Even though she would give anything for me to go back to writing poems and cultural pieces, I always end up giving her to read the dirty things I write today in order to hide my sappy side. Back at home after the clinic, I started looking through one of my trunks again. Finally, I found the yellowing piece of paper, jaundice-colored. It was a letter that my mother had written to me in utero while she was pregnant. Now she believed in the Virgen de las Manzanas, the Andean Apus, and Deepak Chopra, but in those days when she was carrying me in her belly, she was a die-hard union leader who fought alongside my father in some leftist political party and I was the seed of that revolutionary love, merely an idea to believe in, another utopia:

The letter said:

Son or daughter:

Your parents are political, they are policy makers, but things aren't easy on this front, as we'll explain; I'll tell you that this quest is what drives and marks our lives. Forgive us, then, if the emotional tension, the burdens and anger that men and women of action must suffer, have affected you. But we don't want you to be a sad boy or girl; your father and I are not sad either. We know, and you will have felt this, that there are times when we behave like children, we fool around, we laugh, it makes us happy to see a lovely flower whose shape and color give us a feeling of sweetness. I hope that you will experience many more of these moments than solely the ones we give to you. But do you know what should make you truly happy? That neither your dad nor your mom live a bland life; we are passionate, we cannot tolerate injustice or treachery and, especially, cowardice. What will you be like, my son or daughter . . . ?

In my mother's letter full of idealism, affirmation, and hope, I am the only question mark.

At night, I limped to her room and got in her bed. She was asleep. I whispered in her ear or dreamed that I was whispering: "This is how I am, Mom, it doesn't make me happy to look at a flower, I'm not a woman of action but I'm not sad either."

She woke me up very early to do my physical therapy exercises, which consisted of bouncing on an enormous ball. I don't know what, but something didn't hurt so much anymore.

And that's how I lost my sovereignty and, from that moment on, gave myself over completely to the game of being hers once again.

The bad part was that we didn't have much time left. In three days, I was going back to Spain. Once again, out of her strawberry patch forever.

5

APRIL

THE ROUTE FROM the El Prat Airport to Barcelona is along a typical highway on the outskirts of everything. Passing through proliferating industrial parks, it's so anodyne that it could well be the highway that links a person to their final destination. Sitting in the back seat, J and I looked at the city we were about to reclaim. It was a pleasant feeling. Being from one country but living in another is like having a lover without having completely renounced your old, dedicated husband. If one of them fails you, there's always the other one, and vice versa: an official country and a back-up country. Though the paradox was seeing Peru like a summer fling and Spain like the husband who picks you up at the airport without flowers and full of suspicion. As opposed to the eloquent Peruvian taxi drivers, the one from here was content not to utter a single word to us and with that, we could consider ourselves welcomed back. Such coldness might have seemed off-putting at another time, but that day we were grateful for it, as we sat in mute astonishment at everything that suddenly surrounded us once again. As though we were arriving for the first time. I was trying not to look back. When you've heard too many times that children are the hope for tomorrow and, suddenly, you've become the receptacle for that tomorrow, it's easier to think about the future.

The scenery began to look more and more familiar, filling up with identical buildings with the lovely, rusting balconies and waving, sun-faded green awnings typical of apartment buildings in Barcelona. A ray of light cut through a cloud and struck me in the face. I was afraid that it would be traumatic to return to a timid European winter's end with the heat of the southern hemisphere still inside us. But no. I had left a frigid Barcelona and returned to one seized by the fragrant brightness of spring. It put me in a stupendously good mood. In fact, I was happy. There was another reason: though I was still unemployed, we'd be able to pay the rent. J had gotten a new job with a literary magazine.

When we were only a few miles from home, I thought I noticed a flutter inside my stomach which, at first, I attributed to the airplane food. I felt it again and then I knew for sure.

"I think it moved," I said to J.

J put his damp hand on my belly. He felt it too. It was moving. It seemed like a joke. Yet another of the great milestones of pregnancy that left me at a complete loss for words. Once again, an aspiring mother's powers of imagination put to the test and coming up short. These things require new exercises in enunciation. We're dogged always by the same questions: What does it feel like? Like butterfly wings? A caress from inside you? A little viper biting your intestinal tract? Best to stay quiet.

Between eighteen and twenty-two weeks, I remembered, the fetus's movements become perceptible. Mine, for some strange reason, had chosen the precise moment of our return to give us a sign of life. Probably, with all the hubbub in Lima, I hadn't been still enough to notice its vibrations. My accelerated pace had prevented it from expressing itself. Only in those first few moments of calm had it managed to make its presence felt. What was it trying to tell us with its silent dance in the dark? That it felt at ease? That it was home? No one was waiting to greet me at the El Prat airport, just that kick in the stomach.

J got the suitcases out of the taxi, including the heavy one filled with baby clothes that had put an end, once and for all, to our adorable lightness of being. Pushing through my limp, I ran up the stairs. From the balcony, the Sagrada Familia rose, exultant, above the dozens of Japanese tourists who clogged up the sidewalks in that neighborhood. Now that Lima was behind me, I had returned to the subtle reclusion of my small, two-bedroom apartment in Barcelona in which I would have to raise a child, to the sudden gloominess of the skies and the fastidious routine of sweeping up my long hairs that fell to the floor every day. Okay, there's no need to exaggerate. I hadn't arrived, pregnant, on a little boat. I was just another privileged, educated, South American who would have to get in line once a year to renew her tenuous residency, one of those immigrant women who lives in a rented burrow that costs more than an oceanfront apartment in Lima, without a job, without a mother—or may I have, or help yourself, or water, as Vallejo would say. And now with a child waiting in the wings who will inherit this strange way of living. What was I doing here, why did I stay, what was I hoping for in all of this?

We lay down on the bed, looking up at the ceiling and that damp stain we'd never worried about before and said, almost in unison:

"We have to get that fixed."

Spring. It's not wrong what they say. Some pregnant women, well into the second trimester, grown accustomed to our rounded bodies and enormous breasts, think about nothing but sex. It's true that I was worried about finding a job as soon as possible. If I didn't, I wouldn't be able to complete the six months of work that I needed in order to take maternity leave and put my papers in order, but I exorcised my anxiety by getting lost in the galleries of images of naked pregnant women on the Web.

For a more or less heterosexual woman, seeing other women's bodies is also very exciting; seeing tits and vaginas turns us on than seeing an erect penis. I started taking photos of myself. Like I said: I had a lot of free time on my hands. I would get my little digital camera and take pictures of myself in gynecological poses. I dove into hunting for photos of other pregnant women. I thought that only I, and other bulbous women, would be curious about pregnant women's bodies. I was wrong. I discovered an underworld revolving around so-called "belly bumps," which was a subgenre under "bizarre pleasures," alongside zoophilia, obese women, and the elderly. Apparently pregnant women were a pornographic species in themselves, called "nine moons." What could be so exciting for a man about a woman expecting a baby? With our gigantic tits crowned with a pair of dark nipples and the taut skin of our bellies webbed with stretch marks, with our angelic faces and that bountiful glimmer in our eyes, future mothers were seen as literal sex bombs. Somewhere, being pregnant was an erotic plus. I was in luck.

The titles of the photos or videos of expecting women revealed the same creativity as normal porno tapes: "fucking in her last month of pregnancy," "hot mama with tasty pussy," "pregnant woman wants you to watch," "two pregnant lesbians get it on." In the classified listings I found many men seeking pregnant women with whom to live out their fantasies. They offered "economic support" and promised to "spoil them." One said: "I know that pregnant women burn with desire but are too shy to admit it." Another: "They're soooooo delicate." Yet another: "They're more sensitive . . . down below." And so, in the imagination of men partial to pregnant women, we were helpless and horny beings with huge breasts. In short: the ideal woman. One man confessed that he'd been obsessed with having sex with a pregnant woman ever since his wife had kept him on a sexual diet of bread and water during the nine months of her pregnancy: "She didn't like to be touched, her breasts hurt, she felt fat, her head hurt, my cologne bothered her." I found other explanations: not having to use a condom was the stupidest; that it was a way of having a threesome was the most unsettling. Someone posed this question to the forum: "Doesn't it turn you on that someone has already fucked them properly?"

Another threw more fuel on the fire: "What gets me off is knowing that someone fucked her without a condom and came inside her. That drives me wild." Finally, one forum user calling himself "Doctor Dou" maintained: "After the sixth month, pregnant women tend to experience rectal-anal tenesmus (a feeling of emptiness between the anus and rectum), an intense throbbing that they have a tremendous urge to suffocate by taking something completely inside them in that zone, and further, because of hormones, the anal-rectal muscles become distended, inviting deep and sustained intercourse."

There was something to all of this, but the truth is that not all of us have the same luck. Some pregnant women's libidos are very low, either because they worry about hurting the baby or because they're unhappy with the weight gain, and they feel uncomfortable and not the least bit sensual. Also, desire fluctuates throughout the three trimesters, from less to more and from more to less. At first, the nausea and general malaise diminish desire; toward the fourth month, energy returns and desire skyrockets.

That's what was happening to me. Just the night before—because I was too lazy to get up to turn on the computer and go find a porno DVD, and because I would have felt bad waking up J, who was asleep after a long day at work—I had done it in pathetic fashion with the valiant help of my realistic penis-shaped black vibrator, but watching local television channel 25, which airs horrible porn all night long, generally on a tiny screen overrun with ads and scenes that cut off painfully right at the best part.

As pregnancy progresses and the birth approaches, desire recedes again. Sometimes, the problem is not the pregnant woman, but rather her husband. I logged on to a chat room and there was a woman whose husband wouldn't make love to her for fear of injuring the baby: "But my hormones don't understand that and I masturbate multiple times every day and try to be with my lover as often as I can in order to satiate my desire." A pregnant woman with a lover. Now that was hot, way more so than her masturbation sessions. When I was about to leave, the unsatisfied girl messaged me:

"Hi . . . who are you?"

"I'm G. I'm pregnant too."

"Oh, OK. Do you have photos?"

"Uh . . . yes. Do you?"

"I just posted a photo of me. If you send me one of you, I'll send you one of me where you can see my face."

In the photo, the woman, naked, and about seven months pregnant, was lying down, posing somewhere outdoors. I posted one of the more modest photos I'd taken: me in black underwear. In exchange, she showed me three more photos, this time with her face visible, a very normal and very serious face. She was faintly red-haired, even her pubic hair. I called J to come share in the sexual chat room experience with a pregnant lady. J liked it, but he told me that it was most likely a scam in order to get more photos and post them on the Internet. I laughed. I kept chatting with my pregnant colleague, but then we hit a dead end.

"Do you have a webcam?" she asked me.

"No."

"Bye then. I won't do anything without a webcam."

And she logged off. She just left me hanging there.

And still there are people who think that all pregnant women are delicate.

On the day of Sant Jordi, there are literary festivals on every street corner. This is the third year I've participated in this huge Catalan festival celebrating readers and, especially, book sales. The alleyways in Barcelona fill up with bookstalls and the plazas with pro-reading fairs and events. For their part, publishing houses, newspapers, and magazines put on shindigs at which you'll find writers from all over the globe signing books, having a few drinks, and making fools of themselves. In previous years, I had arrived punctually at several of these fairs, accompanied by Ana. I don't know which were more sophisticated, her literary tastes or her methods of seduction, but, in any case, she was perfect company for those utter snobfests. We would begin our Sant Jordi at the party thrown by the newspaper *El Mundo*, then move on to the party in honor of the prize given by the magazine *Qué leer*, and end up at some small, champagne-drenched reception organized by an independent publisher or literary agency in the hippest bar in El Borne, generally surrounded by second-tier journalists and writers whom Ana tended to insult. The next day, we would dance until dawn at the banquet hosted by the publishing house *Planeta* in some sleazy nightclub.

But this year, something had changed. To start with, I'd decided to go to only one party, two at the most. Though I still felt energetic and game to go out, I wasn't up for continuous parties. With only my single allotted glass of wine or the two beers that I drank when I went out, I would never be able to last through one of those interminable parties. I decided that, since it started early, I'd go to the *Qué leer* party at the Ritz, and I'd focus on eating. That was when I opened my closet and came face to face with reality: not a single one of my dresses fit me. I couldn't even get any of them up over my hips or down over my breasts. Since my first great expansion, I'd been wearing loose-fitting, summery clothes, especially in Peru, but since returning to Spain, I'd been living in my pajamas and hadn't even thought of going shopping at one of those maternity-wear places. In fact, I'd decided that I would never wear XXL clothing, and especially not that tacky stuff made just for pregnant women. I preferred to wear wide-legged pants and tight t-shirts that showed off my ample curves and displayed the little marsupial. With my big belly, I thought it was sexy to show off my belly button, and I don't think I'd ever exposed it more brazenly. Later I discovered that I hadn't invented this style and that I belonged to the group who "showed it," as opposed to those with the opposite tendency: those who "hid it." Two ways of being pregnant "that oscillated between comfort and a desire to seduce," according to the guide that seemed to have a horrible sentence at the ready for almost every occasion. At that time, it was stylish to show off your belly, so my intuition hadn't led me astray.

I couldn't wear one of my sexy-pregnant-chick-at-home outfits to go to the Ritz. That was a fact. Anything I might put on would make me look like what I was: a heart-warming pregnant lady. And I could think of no image less appropriate for one of those parties. In desperation,

I called Mica, my loyal friend and style expert, who came to the rescue with some of her most cherished clothes and accessories. We spent a long time trying different combinations, until I realized that J, impeccably dressed, was standing by the door, looking at his watch. The crisis had come to a head.

"Let's go."

"I'm not going."

"You'll regret it later if you don't."

And I didn't go. I'd regret it the next day, but at that moment, stretched out on the couch, eating sunflower seeds and watching TV with Mica, I felt relieved. Something was changing. Either I had to go out and buy clothes that I would never in my life wear again (all pregnant women harbor the hope that we'll return to our pre-pregnancy weight and go back to wearing all the clothes now resting comfortably in the closet), or I'd temporarily retire from nightlife requiring me to be dressed to the nines. I opted for the latter. It wasn't going to kill me to miss a couple of parties. The phone rang. It was Ana, or, more precisely, writer X, who was calling on Ana's behalf to ask me to please bring some deodorant because my friend had forgotten to put any on. I told this person to tell her that I wasn't coming. Ana called me a few minutes later.

"Where the hell are you?"

"At home. I'm not going."

"Why not?!!"

"Because I don't have anything to wear."

"Don't be an ass. Wear your green dress!"

"I can't get it on."

"Oh my God, if you want, we can go to my house and look for something."

"Forget it. I'll call you later. Have a good time."

My social life was taking a nosedive. The next day, I invited a group of friends over for dinner on the terrace, which was the only nice thing about our shitty little apartment. With summer almost upon us, and calculating that I was going to spend the next several months inside that house, we had just bought a table and chairs, an umbrella, and a lounge chair. J and I had spent the morning cleaning and doing a necessary book purge. They sent books to J at the magazine every week, and we were living practically buried in the latest publications. The baby would arrive in a few months and we had to make room for it. I set up a little stand like the ones on La Rambla during Sant Jordi, with books and red roses. We had a barbecue and gave away our books. From then on, I was going to settle for daytime events, preferably those involving a lot of food. As I said: my social life was taking a nosedive.

During an uncomplicated pregnancy there should be three ultrasounds: the first, between the sixth and twelfth weeks, to confirm the pregnancy; the second, between the sixteenth and twentieth weeks, to detect any fetal malformations, and the third at thirty-two weeks to monitor fetal growth. I was about to go in for the second ultrasound, during which we could also find out the baby's sex.

I had reached twenty weeks, and that gave me the right to find out if I was expecting a girl or a boy, unless it was a particularly modest or mischievous baby, in which case it would hide its shame with some strange pose, occasionally even up until the day of its birth.

There are parents, not many, but they do exist, who choose not to learn their baby's sex. These strange beings believe in a return to natural ways, to the days before ultrasounds existed and people laid bets about whether it was a girl or a boy. At the other extreme are the no less strange parents who want to know immediately so they can give it a name and so they never call it "the baby," but Jimena or Sebastián instead. And they talk about him or her as if they were there next to them, and they practically set a place at the table for them and make you greet them by name when you go over for a visit. These people also think it's best to find out so they know whether to buy blue or pink baby clothes.

As for me, I was pretty tired of having to constantly take a side in one stupid controversy or another. In the world of absolute uncertainty in which pregnant women live, everything becomes a matter of State. We are so easily manipulated it's disgusting. We listen to our mothers, our mothers-in-law, our cousins, our friends, and they all say different things and we believe them all. Our heads are like balls of wool. I was trying to listen only to a few of them. For example, my Basque friend, Aixi. Before, she had been an unrelenting traveler who thought it very unlikely that she'd have a baby in this lifetime. But now she had a beautiful two-month-old daughter. Aixi's natural temperament led her to adopt a militant position about almost everything. When I was with her, maternity seemed not only a natural act, but also a political one: deciding to bottle-feed your baby would define you, committing you to a particular path and its repercussions. If you put your baby in a stroller you're one kind of mother, but if you wear it strapped to your body in a sling you're another. You have to decide if you'll be one of those obedient mothers who rigorously follows the vaccination schedule because your pediatrician tells you to, or one who believes that vaccines are inventions by huge laboratories seeking to enrich themselves at our children's expense. What do you choose? Will you take your baby to the pediatrician? Will you use anti-stretch mark cream or prickly pear seed oil? Will you apply nipple cream or use your own milk to soothe cracked nipples? Will the baby sleep in your room, in your bed, or will it have its own room? Will you pick it up when it cries or will you let it cry it out so it doesn't become spoiled? Will you choose a birth with or without anesthesia? Will you insist they put the baby on your chest right after it is born or will you let them take it away to clean it up first? Will your husband cut the umbilical cord or will he stick to taking photos? Will you let them give you an oxytocin drip to accelerate labor or will you want a labor that lasts forty-eight hours? Will you let them cut your perineum or will you protest? Will you give your baby mashed solid food before six months or only milk? Boy or girl? Take a side, take a side, take a side!!!

The baby's sex as aesthetic determinant. All women who have been mothers think themselves a bit of an oracle. The majority of mothers I came across told me that they could "tell by my face that it was going to be a girl." I've heard this theory dozens of times: being pregnant with a girl makes you ugly because the baby steals the mother's beauty; being pregnant with a boy makes you beautiful because it just does. The worst part is that I've also heard the inverse theory just as often: beautiful if you're expecting a girl and ugly if you're expecting a boy. Another myth to hack to pieces. It goes without saying that, no matter what sex the baby is, if you have a difficult pregnancy, if you're vomiting and suffering from constant, horrible pain, you can be sure that you're not going to want to ask the mirror who is the most beautiful one of all in the kingdom. Now if, on the other hand, you feel fantastic and people pay an unusual amount of attention to you, you'll start to feed off of this heightened interest and respond to it by taking more care with your appearance than usual. The difference is between a fucked-up pregnancy and a not-fucked-up pregnancy. That, for the moment, was my only hypothesis.

All pregnancy guides have, of course, a chapter called "Beauty During Pregnancy." The advice is fascinating. You must take as a point of departure, they say, that when one's silhouette expands it's very difficult to feel seductive. All I could think of was that Maitena cartoon (and when I think of a Maitena cartoon it's because something's not going well) in which she describes two types of pregnant women: the sexy pregnant woman who, despite her sweet little belly, retains her statuesque figure but adds a new pair of tits, provoking appreciative cries of "Oh, mama!" as she passes by; and the refrigerator-shaped pregnant woman, who also provokes cries of "Oh, mama!," except these are uttered in terror.

One book recommends taking advantage of the resplendent skin typical of a pregnant woman by using only simple, natural makeup. I know women who've had discolored patches bloom and hair sprout on their faces during pregnancy, so that advice isn't for everyone. Another recommendation is to wear fresh-smelling perfumes and fragrances, as "pregnant women sweat a lot," a new euphemism that means pregnant ladies' armpits stink. I closed the book and went to take a bath.

I don't know if this information that I found on a specialized website had any scientific basis, but it certainly sounded absurd.

You're expecting a boy if:
— Fetal heart rate is under 140 beats per minute.
— You're carrying low and your belly is pointy in shape.
— Your urine is a crystal-clear yellow color.
— Your right breast is more swollen than your left.
— You didn't experience any morning sickness during the first trimester of your pregnancy.

On the other hand, you're expecting a girl if:
— Fetal heart rate is over 140 beats per minute.
— You're carrying high and your belly is rounded.
— Your urine is clear.
— Your left breast is more swollen than your right.
— You sleep on your left side.

As for my answers to the quiz: my belly was not low or pointy, but high and rounded. My urine might have been a little bit yellow, but nothing out of the ordinary. The breast thing was even more complicated because they looked the same to me. The last part was unsettling: I had experienced nausea during the first trimester. Add to this that people were constantly commenting on how beautiful I looked. Were they lying, or was I having a girl?

I had returned home.

I had taken out the trash.

I had drunk a glass of cold milk and splattered the floor with white drops.

I was alone. Slowly, I had organized, yet again, the folder in which I was keeping all the recent paperwork about my pregnancy. The folder that contained the last days of my life or the first of someone else's. Suddenly, my history was the history of *another*. My pregnant-lady card on which my data were recorded was in there, along with the images from the second ultrasound I'd just had. One of them was of a big head in silhouette with one hand extended. The other was a close-up of its genitalia.

That afternoon, the doctor and his intern were waiting for me, ready to conduct a practical lesson in high-resolution ultrasound. It was obvious that I was to be their guinea pig. Once again, I was surprised at how doctors can live completely on the margins of people and their stories, talking the whole time about organs and body parts, always in their own, complex language, interacting only with their peers and making you feel like an unwanted guest in a scene from your own life. The distance between that and unlawful sterilization was only a few short steps. I once read that, around 1971, an institute was founded in Los Angeles where women were taught to look inside their own vaginas with a speculum and a mirror. It made a lot of sense to not have to depend on health professionals for all our internal matters, especially those related to sex and reproduction.

The sonographer seemed to be very experienced and was explaining everything to the bespectacled intern, who was peering into my innards as if they were a PlayStation.

"Do you see the difference?" the sonographer was saying. "This woman is a primigravida. Look at the shape of her uterus."

Apparently, this was a lesson in Comparative Sonography. He smeared my belly with gel and as he moved the wand over me, I could see the fetus, with its disproportionate head and shrunken body. It had changed since the last time. The doctor, looking at the black-and-white screen, began tallying up organs, confirming that all extremities were present and accounted for. That there were lungs, that the heart was properly situated, that the skull had grown sufficiently, that the kidneys and the liver were functioning well. Public hospitals don't tend to use 3D and 4D technology because they are very expensive systems and traditional ultrasound is almost equally effective. One of those kinds of ultrasounds can cost you up to 180 euros in a private clinic. Any charlatan with one of those devices and zero medical training could make a killing offering photos and videos during pregnancy. I had to content myself with the modest, flat, somewhat antiquated yet reliable view of my firstborn. In that pathetic image, I couldn't even tell if he or she was photogenic.

"What is it, a boy or a girl?" I asked anxiously.

"Wait a minute. Right now we're looking at more important things."

For these solemn doctors, the matter of the baby's sex was of secondary concern. It was akin to the sensationalist news item of the day, the one newspapers use as a headline not for its importance, but rather for its impact. The truly important thing is that, thanks to this diagnostic procedure, it would be possible to detect the principal fetal malformations. It is known that between three and six percent of babies will have an anomaly (of this percentage, up to twelve percent will be chromosomal anomalies or genetic abnormalities, though, since these can't be detected through ultrasound, it is necessary to perform other kinds of diagnostic tests). These could be problems relating to blood circulation between the fetus and the mother or problems with the baby's morphological structure. If these defects are incompatible with life, the decision can be made at that point to interrupt the pregnancy.

"Now then, we can clearly see that it's a girl. There's no doubt about it."

Well, I had been liberated from the thorny decision about whether or not to circumcise. I had already decided I wouldn't pierce her ears. After the trauma of being born, why would I receive you with a wound?

Monday, April 24, 2006.

Dear X:

We had returned home.

Yes, now we were alone, just the two of us. I'm not exactly a chatterbox, especially not with people who can't (or don't want) to answer me. This, in fact, is something you'll appreciate in the future. Anyway, you don't need me to open my mouth, you're content with the sounds my body and my heart make and with the fact that I'm alive. I'm content that, every once in a while, you kick me from the inside.

I just wanted to tell you that it's lucky that you weren't born a hundred years ago, and definitely better than two hundred years ago, better for you and me both, obviously. And that we don't live, for example, in Iran or Ciudad Juárez. Because if any of that were the case, my beloved daughter, you would not have been good news. You would have been an explicit call to insurrection.

I'm writing to you because I have something very concrete to tell you. I used to think of you as one of those household bugs that live out their lives unseen right in the middle of the living room; but today I saw you and I think you waved at me. Ergo: you are not a bug. You are much more than a bug. Ever since I found out that I was pregnant I've called you "*bebito*." I suppose it was a neutral enough term of address, but the truth is that hidden within it was my wish that you'd be a boy. I was afraid of the psychological pitfalls inherent in having a child of the same sex. A bunch of nonsense they teach you in college. Now, suddenly, I needed to wrap my head around the idea that you are a baby girl.

What's more problematic for me is calling someone *her* that I've always referred to as *him*, more or less like when a friend decides to change their sex. You'll understand one day. Kisses. See you soon.

Today, a woman with a certain postfeminist bent has the option of being a little of everything: she can use contraceptives and postpone motherhood, she can abort in the case of carelessness or mental confusion. She can get married or cohabitate, be an economist or a housewife, or both at the same time. But she can also choose, instead of giving birth in a hospital, to do so at home and in the water, with the help of a midwife, remaining coherent the whole time. She can have a baby and quit her job as a high-level executive in a multinational corporation in order to spend more time with said baby. A liberated woman and the ideal mother. Can she do it all?

For my part, I was having problems seeing myself as a postfeminist. I had signed up with a Catalonian government employment agency, but no one had called me. No one wanted a pregnant woman. We are anti-aesthetic beings in the labor world. I wasn't surprised. But at least I'd be able to prove to the government when I went to renew my residency that I hadn't been working, not because I didn't want to, but because no one would hire me. But this didn't free me from having to find a job as soon as possible. I needed to pay into social security for a while longer in order to have the right to claim benefits during the four months that, by law, I was going to care for my baby at home.

I had to turn to my friends. It didn't seem like such a big deal to me, but to judge by their faces when I told them my story, my case was pretty pitiful, and many of them took an interest and told me they'd let me know if they heard of anything. In the first world, the majority of people get pregnant only after they've already picked out schools for their kids, not when they have absolutely nothing going for them. I was on the verge of signing on as an editorial assistant at a small publishing house that had offered me a three-month contract, but without a salary and through which I'd have to pay into social security myself, but luckily it didn't pan out. I was brimming with desperation. Finally, I got a call from an ex-colleague at the now-defunct magazine *Lateral*, and she told me that her brother-in-law worked for a veterinary association and they needed someone who could sit for six hours a day and enter the names of dogs and cats, along with their corresponding chip numbers, into a gigantic database. Once, I was a journalist who, during her early days in Barcelona, had had to climb a mountain carrying a heavy backpack filled with flyers from a pizzeria called Sapri and go door to door stuffing mailboxes, terrified of the outsize hatred that junk mail provoked in people. I had had to wash enormous, greasy paella skillets until my hands peeled, under the yoke of a tremendously fat Moroccan woman who didn't speak a single word of Spanish.

What more could I want? I was moving up in the world.

6

MAY

ONCE AGAIN, life imitates *Second Life* and not the other way around. "Bundle of Joy" is the name of the maternity clinic in that parallel world, the place an avatar wanting to get pregnant needs to visit. In this virtual fertility store it's possible to purchase a belly for 500 Linden Dollars and, for much less, some fabulous maternity clothing. You can buy babies there, too. Everyone can get pregnant, men and women, and you can choose your little one's skin and eye color, and even its species: anthropomorphic, cyborg, etc. An avatar who couldn't have children invented the SL maternity clinic, thinking she could also help others like her. The advantages are obvious: the gestation period lasts only twenty-one days, you can abort legally and without remorse or physical discomfort. Ditto for the delivery and, as if that weren't enough, if, after being born, the offspring turns out to be a nuisance, you can simply archive it and go about

your life. But I, damn the luck, exist in the realm of the
first life, though, actually, it's not all that different. The
flesh and blood avatars I keep coming across are also
customized and they've done much worse things in order
to have children. They've had a second chance to live out
the lives they wanted to live.

What causes a person to yearn to become a mother/
father even in cases in which it goes against their own
nature, exposing them to incomprehension and social
isolation? How in the hell does our biological clock work?
Who puts in the batteries or takes them out?

"MY BUNDLE OF JOY"

AVATAR: GEMMA
APPEARANCE: CURLY BLACK HAIR. GLASSES. BLUE JACKET.

I'm the fashion designer with premature menopause
who hung posters in universities offering 800 euros
for a young woman's eggs. I'm the one who joined an
internet forum and discovered that there are girls who'll
exchange their eggs for money. I'm the one who got a
call from Alelí, a blond twenty-year-old who worked
cleaning stairwells. She offered me her eggs and, in so

doing, became the last, best hope that my family tree wouldn't turn into a withered twig. In return for Alelí's eggs, the hospital gave me some other eggs from an anonymous woman. Before all of this, I'd been feeling like an old hen laying hollow eggs. Well, it's not like I think my blood will turn to poison if I don't have a child, but it's just naive to believe that, in the twenty-first century, there are still some things that are impossible, don't you think? That's why I tried it. I want fresh eggs from fertile girls, sweet, viable little strangers' eggs I can use as though they were mine, eggs that, in the wee hours of the night, will be lovelessly combined with my husband's semen in a sterile test tube. Immaculate conception through artificial insemination. Without sex, without pleasure, exchanging the bedroom for the laboratory. One day I cried out in horror at the looming biological desert, and I told myself that I would pay any amount to get pregnant. Philip Roth, a writer I read often, has a good explanation for this business of having children: we have them in order to hear something in between our moans of sexual pleasure and our death rattles. Personally, during this ellipsis, I want to hear a baby's cry. I don't want a little Chinese girl found in a ditch. That's fine for Angelina Jolie. I don't need anyone to know how good I am or how good everyone's been to me. I want to give birth to a baby and maybe, one day, tell him the truth about his origins, tell him about the blond girl who cleaned stairwells. I want to nurse him—just like a mother elephant might nurse a baby hyena in a hypothetical *National Geographic* documentary—I want to nurse that child interloper, that hybrid result of my husband's genes and the genes from that other woman's eggs, the child who will not have my snub nose, or my faraway look, or my sad smile. I want to harbor him for nine obese months, for him to be tethered to me, to feed him food that I chew myself, to quit smoking on his behalf, to teach him to listen to the murmur of the Mediterranean and to give birth to him in a bloody scene, preferably recorded on home video. I want an irrational love. But you should also know that the last treatment didn't go well. They discovered that the neck of my uterus is very narrow. Another of Mother Nature's jokes. Another challenge for Sister Science. My child waits, frozen, for the climate to improve. I know that soon I'll be able to tell him the day and the exact hour of his conception, something that other children cannot know. I'll tell him that I saw the beginning of life on a screen, the beginning of his life, like in a science fiction movie. He'll like that, don't you think?

AVATAR: ALELÍ

APPEARANCE: BLOND, TALL, 19 YEARS OLD, BLUE EYES,
  COTTON CLOTHING.

Not long ago, someone stole my bicycle because I'd left it
chained to a tree overnight. Incredibly, three days later, while
I was drinking a Coca-Cola with a friend on Barceloneta
Beach, I saw my old bicycle zoom by, painted an electric
blue. It was several miles away from where it had been
stolen! There are things that come back to you for some
reason, I suppose because you love them so much, and
there are things that don't come back, and you just have
to forget them, allow them to be lost forever. Do I believe
that one day a familiar-seeming twenty-year-old boy will
knock on my door and, when I serve him a cup of coffee,
he'll accidentally spill it on the tablecloth just like I do
every morning? I ask you: what would you do if a woman
you didn't know from Eve turned up on a talk show swear-
ing to be your "real" mother? Isn't that reason enough not
to watch those kinds of programs? Well, whatever. Why
think about these things? It doesn't do any good.

You tell me I'm too good-hearted and positive, an altru-
istic being. Well, it's true, I am. You ask me if I feel an
insane curiosity, a morbid fascination, if a ghost circles
around me at night. And how can I make you understand

that the money is just an incentive, that my true feeling is that I'm doing something good in order to earn it. Many people accuse me of selling children. But I'm not going to carry them inside me! In fact, if I don't donate them, I'll get my period and they'll just go straight down the drain.

I think I'm as anxious as Gemma to see that baby, or even more so. I hope to be like an auntie to it. Gemma and I became inseparable in the hospital, when we had to get injections together at the same time, and ever since then, she's been like a second mother to me.

What is a mother? For me, she's most like a giantess who smells of milk, a lioness with a brain, vampire fangs, mermaid eyes and a mouth like Plato's cave.

The eight hundred euros are great, but I'll still be taking care of old people and scrubbing staircases, and, God willing, one day I'll study interior design.

AVATAR: ALE

APPEARANCE: 5'2." DARK HAIR. COLORFUL CLOTHING.

I'm a future single mother even though the father is dying to be part of the plan. In Lima I was a stage actress, but in Barcelona I work in a bar. I don't want anything in my life that enslaves me. I do what I want and that's that. I don't care about success or recognition, or about doing great things. There are plenty of people doing that already. For me, having free time and being able to enjoy it is the most valuable thing. The world isn't lacking for better professionals or better artists but rather, better human beings. Why would I want an impressive job if it would just end up taking over my entire life? I'm the type who lets life surprise me. I'm 33 and I guess my biological clock went off. Three years ago I aborted a baby that I had wanted, driven by common sense rather than emotion. I still didn't have my papers, the father of that baby wasn't even in Barcelona and our relationship was uncertain. For a pragmatic person, it wasn't a viable option. I never forgave myself for not being brave enough to risk it; it was something I owed to myself. That potential father disappeared and, shortly after, I fell in love with (and am still in love with) a guy who definitely does not want to have a baby because he already has one. Since I couldn't make him change his mind, I decided to go my own way. I threw myself into "operation baby." It took no time at all. No sooner had I embarked on the operation than I was already happily impregnated by a wild, young street musician who was kind enough to understand where I was coming from and to collaborate in an efficient and unselfish way. The first month I was pretty freaked out, hysterical, I didn't want to see anyone, I felt weird and disoriented and even my very closest friends were incredibly annoying to me. I was a total downer. That's the truth. Now I'm happy. Of course, it's hard to juggle work and everything else, but it's worth it. I don't have much of a sex drive these days, even though before I was a real champ in that arena. I'm no longer with the father; he was just a collaborator, our sexual relations had been for breeding purposes only. Although we still cuddle and fool around a bit, there's no penetration, and I think this helps me psychologically to disengage from him. Despite the pregnancy, my ex and I still have a certain sexual connection, though obviously it's become tender and cautious, with none of the wildness of before. So sex isn't a problem. Aside from the economics, the biggest challenge of doing this alone is not being able to share responsibilities. I have to handle everything, or almost everything, on my own. Theoretically, it's easier with two people, but the advantage of doing it alone is that there are no conflicts. There's something else I'm discovering: not having a partner doesn't mean that you're completely alone. There's a whole web of relationships. I'm surprised at how pampered I am. I don't have a partner to take care of me but I have five or six people looking out for me. I'm only four months pregnant right now. I don't know what will happen later. I'm Ale and I'm not alone.

AVATAR: MARIBEL

APPEARANCE: 38 YEARS OLD. WHITE. BLUE EYES. THIN.

I've never been like Susanita (that little girl in the *Mafalda* comic strip) who dreamed her whole life of having babies. I'm an anthropologist, so (occupational hazard) I believe in constructs, in cultural relativity and all that stuff, but I was also born within a family, within a social and cultural framework. I was married to a man, which is more or less what was expected of me, as was the assumption that I would have children. When I met Tati, when I accepted everything that being with Tati meant, the discovery, the freedom, the totality of giving myself over, there was a perhaps implicit renunciation, or at least a postponement, of the idea of having a child. Our life together was all-encompassing. Being with her was more important than any thought of a future baby. Then we came to Spain. In Lima, we had opened up some space for ourselves, but it was still like a big closet. I remember the first time we went to a gay pride march in Barcelona. There were a ton of people marching with the slogan "Equality Now," and they were demanding the right to marry. I was amazed. Despite everything I'd been through, I suddenly thought: It's possible, we can ask for this. More than discovering our rights, it was about realizing to what extent we still didn't accept ourselves. Within that context, Tati and I started planning to be mothers.

For me, wanting to be a mother has been, first and foremost, a process of recuperating that old desire and also something that emerges powerfully as part of a couple. Our daughter is the product of the two of us as a couple, much beyond what one might conventionally believe. Different from other couples in which only one partner wants to be pregnant, in our case we both wanted to have that experience, so we decided that we'd each have a baby. We decided that Tati should go first because she was a little older than me.

I put a lot of thought into the idea of bonding. I worked hard to achieve it. Not only because we were two moms, but because I was a non-biological mom. The other day, a friend of mine was talking about pregnancy and she said that it was too bad that men missed out on the experience, and it sounded so strange to me because I wasn't pregnant and, nevertheless, I experienced Tati's pregnancy as though it were mine.

When our daughter was born, it was like coming out of the closet all over again. Now the whole world would know: the baker, the cashier at the supermarket, the neighbor. We wanted it to be that ordinary. The world is prepared only for one mother and we would have to disabuse it of that notion.

Now I'm the pregnant one and something strange is happening to me: I thought that when it was my turn, I wouldn't have to work at forging the bond, that the bond would be created by the biology, but no, I've realized that you have to create it just the same. I think something similar happens to all mothers with their second child, they think they won't be able to love another child the way they love the first one. It's the same thing.

It was awe-inspiring to witness Tati giving birth, and now I'm going to experience it from the other side. And she will too. I think this is one of those few things that only we lesbians can do.

AVATAR: MARUJA

APPEARANCE: RED HAIR. TALL. DARK EYES.

I took these pills and after ten days a white drop dampened my nipple. I brought him to my breast and told him to suck. He rejected it at first. He'd already been taking a bottle for a while. He would let go of the nipple and I would put it back in his mouth, poking it in there with my finger. His failed attempts made my nipples hurt and start to crack. One day he managed to latch on and he didn't stop. It was so perfect to see my son, with his dark skin, nursing from my feeble white breast. We brought him from Africa. His mother died of AIDS, but luckily did not transmit the virus to him.

I had been trying to get pregnant for over a decade. I always wanted to be a mother. The adoption process was incredibly long and exhausting. I think it's more painful than giving birth. I almost threw in the towel several times before they finally gave us our Certificate of Suitability. As soon as we had that, we started in on all the other paper-work. Like it says in a book I read, we adoptive mothers have pregnancies like elephants—they last for over two years.

The pills I take are called sulpiride, I think, and they induce the production of prolactin and oxytocin, which respond to the stimulus of suction. Induced lactation is the solution for adoptive mothers like me who want to strengthen their bond with their children. We are so different physically that we have to bond in other ways. I don't know if, as some say, this makes me a biological mother, but when he's nursing, our eyes meet and communicate. It's as if we finally belong to each other.

AVATAR: DORA

APPEARANCE: BIG. DIRTY. TANGLED HAIR.

My father killed my mother. He slit her throat because he was a poultry vendor in the Agustino market and he knew how to cut up each piece without leaving any loose bones. I was ten years old, but that day I learned that a human being splatters a thousand times more than a chicken. That's why I'm stained with blood. But it isn't my mother's blood, I don't think. I killed something else—it wasn't a chicken, it was a pig—without a knife. What for, when I've got my hands? My hands are so dirty they inspire fear. It doesn't matter anymore. The fact is I'm here, like inside a rock. Yes, I'm inside a silent rock that's inside a mountain made of tumbling stones. Sometimes I think we'll never be able to fall all the way down to the bottom. Or that this is a bottomless pit. Sometimes freedom scares me more than prison. When they locked me up I didn't know what was happening. When you spend a lot of time on the streets, you forget when you last ate and what it was that you ate. It's the same with the other thing. I don't know how this baby got inside me, I just know that it's growing inside walls, like me, and that the poor thing will be born and will go on being inside walls. At least until it's three years old, when by law, they'll take it from me all over again and toss it into the same streets I came off of. Ever since my belly started to grow, the guards have treated me better, and the prisoners too. Everyone says how clever of you, *china*, to come in here with a baby on board, pregnant inmates get prison benefits, you scored, *gordita*. So many of us are in here missing our kids on Mother's Day and on all the rest of the days too, but you're gonna have him in here with you, to keep you company those nights under that blanket hopping with fleas when you'd give anything to be a noxious gas escaping underneath the door. But I don't know what to say to them. I just put my plate of chicken and rice on top of my big belly as if it were a folding table and tear some shreds of meat off with my teeth, with my dirty hands. We don't use knives in here. When it's born I'll have to teach it to eat like us.

AVATAR: SHEILA
APPEARANCE: TALL. CURLY HAIR. BIG NOSE.

I don't know why it's so hard for people to accept that some of us don't want to be mothers. I don't mean just not right now, but never. I never ever want to be a mother. It's not that I haven't found the perfect man. In fact, I think I have a perfect man by my side and I know it because he agrees with me on this. It's just that I'm not seduced by the idea of becoming a mere receptacle, of deforming my body and dying of pain in a delivery room in order to bring a child into the world who will make my life impossible. I'm not the least bit interested in ceasing to be the center of my own life, the one who gets spoiled at home, or in lavishing a mother's adoration for twenty long years, which is how long it takes for a human child to become independent, and only then because you finally dare to give him a kick in the ass to help him out the door. Why do you think I'm being such a hard-ass about this? I'm not just posturing, I'm thinking clearly. I've watched my sister fuck up her life for her child—let's be clear—for the little dictator she has for a son. She and other mothers live in a permanent state of unacknowledged postpartum depression. I've come to think that the government should put up ads in the street with slogans like "Don't try it," "Just say NO to pregnancy" or "Have good friends, not babies," just like those anti-drug campaigns, but with photos before and after having a baby. Maybe then they'll finally get it.

7

JUNE

I SCHLEPPED every morning to the metro, hauling my heavy, taut belly under the punishing sun, contracting and relaxing my perineum along the way. I got off at Guinardó Station and, from there, walked eight blocks to the office. Coming home from the office, the journey was even more hostile. At two in the afternoon, the sun struck me smack in the face. It was like blushing violently. The sun turned in circles like a ship and came to rest on my head. A small woodpecker emerged from the ship and pecked at my belly as though I were a dead tree trunk from which it was extracting tiny worms with its sharp tongue. I would wake up, keep walking down Passeig de Maragall. I turned into the Boa Constrictor Nebulosa, giving birth to sixty live babies, each four inches long, right there on the pavement. The police stopped traffic, but they gave me a ticket. Next to the metro station sat the Romanian churro vendor, fatter than ever, using her fingers to push the batter into boiling oil, listening to Massiel's "Brindaremos por ti." I opened my eyes and went into the mouth of the metro station, or into the mouth of a time tunnel from which ayahuasca vines hung like strands of drool. Everything grew dark. Inside, J and I and another girl were making love but the baby we'd left sleeping on the floor started crying and we had to stop having sex, get dressed, and hail a taxi. I left the metro station, the light blinding me, and ran into the little old man in the white guayabera shirt and the African prostitute asking him to buy her some cotton candy. White monkeys looked down at us from the trees. In the distance, an old barn caught fire and crows came flying out from inside it. When I was nearly home, I saw the Holy Family appear before me, but suddenly the Holy Family turned into a rusting carousel in the middle of a square, a carousel filled with happy children waving goodbye to me, a carousel that turned into a black octopus that squeezed and squeezed.

I started having something like hallucinations in the middle of my seventh month. It wasn't that I saw angels or elves, but suddenly I'd be inside a daydream that would lead me into another and then another. I suppose it had to do with knowing that I was seven months along and that I was carrying a complete human being, ready to be born. That's why I burst into tears every two seconds. Watching the news or listening to a Dyango song. But also, life wasn't as easy as it had been before; tying my shoes wasn't as easy as it had been before. I was almost at thirty weeks and I had gained a lot of weight. The fetus was now fifteen inches long and weighed nearly four pounds. In just a month, it had doubled its weight. I wasn't sleeping much—lying down was uncomfortable, I was always too hot and I had to get up every two hours to pee. My life oscillated between trying to suck down enough oxygen and trying not to pee my pants. Not to mention the horrendous cramps I suffered in the wee hours of the night that made me suddenly howl with pain. Also while sleeping, I had attacks of the famous Braxton Hicks contractions, practice contractions which, though they don't hurt, do leave you feeling breathless. Your belly grows hard for several moments and it's always a bit scary. Then it passes. Women often confuse them for labor pains. The first time I had strong ones I ran to the doctor thinking I'd gone into labor. After that, I started feeling them up to ten times a day. If they happened while I was walking I had to stop and rest. If they happened while I was making love I had to stop that too. All of this was making me wish more and more that D Day ("d" for delivery) would arrive, and this eagerness made the days seem twice as long. Well, in fact, they were longer because summer was upon us and it stayed light until nine o'clock at night and was incredibly hot twenty-four hours a day. For the past several weeks, the baby had been reacting like a wild goat to my stimuli: my voice, my changes in mood, my tears, the music I put on to help me write: all of it made her move. More and more, I could see her movements from the outside, flesh rising and falling. I would put J's hand on my belly so he could feel the same excitement and we made bets about where her head and her feet were. I felt like she was kicking me in the ribs, just beneath my breasts and between my lungs, which is why I couldn't get enough air at various points throughout the day. If I was out with friends and she started to move, I would go off on my own in order to feel it more clearly. I would make anyone who happened to be next to me hold their hand on my belly until they felt her prancing kicks. At that point, her ears were fully developed. My mother had sent me a CD, *Mozart for Babies*, and my cousin Jessica sent me one with traditional lullabies. My friend Mica had loaned me a set of small speakers and I set them up around my belly. Sometimes, I would neutralize the lullabies with a little punk rock by the Ramones.

—

The baby's name. I read in one of my books: "a name is the first gift we give to our child and also a way of establishing a closer bond with him or her."

Another hurdle along the one-way trip that is pregnancy. A name lasts an entire lifetime. For a task with so much responsibility attached, I could turn to the calendar of saints' days, to mythology, the names of movie stars, rock stars, Nobel Prize winners, royalty, politicians, cities or fictional characters. But why bother choosing so carefully when, in the end, people were just going to call them "Princess" or "Champ," or even worse things?

J was much more paranoid than I was. He was named after his father and he had a younger brother who also had the same name. On top of that, his middle name wasn't a name at all. It was a nominal clause with an alternative spelling formed by two names which his father had combined in a fit of originality, the result being a name one might consider exotic, if one were being kind.

Before we knew we were having a girl, we had two names in mind: Lucas and Mateo. What can I say? Biblical baby names were in fashion. Neither would work now that we were having a girl, obviously, although we tried several variations of Lucas since J had some twisted fantasy of one day saying to our child: "Luke, I am your father," or something like that. We wondered how it would be to name her

Luca, which sounded fairly unisex, even though it was the name of one of the thugs in *The Godfather*. I didn't think it was half bad, but before making up our minds I decided that consulting one of those *Choose Your Baby's Name* books wouldn't make me any more or less cool.

I found the baby name book in our local library. It was one that put a lot of emphasis on the meanings of names. Gabriela, a name of Hebrew origin, meant "woman of God" or "force of God," which correlates with the attributes of the archangel Gabriel, God's messenger and the very one who told Mary of her pregnancy. The natural traits of a person with my name, according to the book, were a person "who seeks attention and feels superior to others, loves experiences, knowledge, and evidence, and likes to feel rewarded." Also, the book went on, a person with my name would "excel in professions such as efficiency expert, manufacturer, executive, businessperson, public employee, banker, or interpreter." Awesome.

Back at home, I discovered that several websites offered search engines for original names. Yes, originality was an option when it came to choosing a name for your baby. In the "baby's sex" field, I wrote: girl. In the "origin" field, I ticked off something that sounded super weird: "Proto-Basque" (there were more of these types of origins: Araucanian, Pseudo-Egyptian, Spanish Hypocorism,

Latin Ecclesiastical). You also had to choose between long and short, classical or original. I chose long and original. Finally, they wanted to know what letter the name should begin with. I put L and pressed enter. No results. I tried other possible combinations and names began to appear: Cloroaldo, Etelvino, Concordio, Andrónico, Prisciliano, Longombardina, Sandalio, and Querubina.

Since originality wasn't working, I moved on to a more conservative website that counseled avoiding original and trendy names at all costs. This site suggested that the crux of the baby name question lay in three questions that should be used, almost blindly, as selection criteria: "Will the name suit the child's personality? Will he or she like the name as an adult? Will it go out of style?" The site proposed names that walked the line between classical, original, and enduring. They were: Valentina, Lara, Sabrina, Juliana, Sofía, Andrea, and Abigail.

From that list, the names we liked were already taken by cousins or friends. The business of choosing a name was transforming from an amusing pastime to a sophisticated form of torture. After many attempts, we each made a list. At the top of my list was Clara, which J considered atrocious. Finally, out of nowhere, came a name that was long, classical, strong, feminine, biblical, and also happened to be the name of the neighborhood in Lima where I'd lived for the better part of my life: Magdalena. But then, almost simultaneously, Lena entered the competition, the name of the main character from Faulkner's *Light in August*, a novel that had deeply affected J and told the story of a pregnant woman named Lena who embarks on a long journey in search of the father of her baby. As an added coincidence, our Lena, if that's what we decided to name her, would be born in August. But Magdalena, although it alluded to the repentant sinner, continued to seem just as good as Lena, so we decided to invent a convoluted formula: we'd name her Magdalena but instead of calling her Magda for short, which we found unbearable, we'd call her Lena, light in August. It all sounded so lovely, it all sounded so poetic, it all sounded like we were up to our eyeballs in this and there was no turning back.

One day I received a call from Eulalia, my midwife. On the last tests they'd done at the end of my sixth month, on something called the O'Sullivan test that measures glucose tolerance, I'd gotten a 173 out of a maximum of 140. This could mean: a) I'd eaten too much bread and jam and it had caused a spike in blood sugar; or b) I had the dreaded gestational diabetes, a type of diabetes that occurs only during pregnancy, especially in mothers over thirty-five and/or with diabetic relatives (in my case, my beloved grandmother). Eulalia was very clear that a genetic predisposition was a much more important factor than the gallon of dulce de leche ice cream I'd eaten over the weekend and the millions of desserts and sweets I'd ravaged since becoming pregnant.

I'd gained only two pounds this month. I weighed 152, which is to say that I was gaining just a bit more than two pounds per month. This was superb. Maybe my belly was a little too big—it was 30 centimeters and 27 was the norm—but it wasn't really something to worry about. In other words, I felt perfect. If it turned out that I'd eaten too much sugar, I would have to rein it in a bit with the chocolate, but in general terms, nothing much would have to change.

On the other hand, if we were talking about gestational diabetes, that is, if I had an excess of sugar in my blood, then there was a very good chance that it would be passed on to the baby through the placenta. She would grow too big and could injure her arms and shoulders coming out of my vagina or require a cesarean section. Her lungs, her liver, everything might function poorly. Lena's organs might not develop completely and there was even the threat of premature labor. After birth, her glucose levels could plummet so low that she'd produce extra insulin, which would force her organs to work harder than normal. This was horrible. I was scared. I would condemn my daughter to prenatal obesity. Suffering would seem an ordinary thing to her, synonymous with life itself.

As for me, the more I learned about gestational diabetes, the more horrified I felt. I, the mother, might also fail to escape high blood pressure, infections, cesarean section, death in childbirth, and that was just for starters. I would also have an increased risk of developing permanent diabetes in the future. This time of "sweet expectation" was beginning to take on an ominous undertone.

To find out if I had diabetes or not, I'd have to undergo another test, this one called "the curve." To prepare for this test, I had to follow a strict diet for three days that almost plunged me into a depression, but there was actually a much worse possibility: if I really had diabetes, I'd have to adhere to this diet for months (and maybe years), and right at the moment I was feeling tremendously hungry. They'd give me a little machine to measure my glucose several times a day and a doctor specializing in gestational diabetes would supervise the entire process.

On the day of "the curve," I had to get up at dawn and, fasting, go to the hospital. For a pregnant woman, the experience of fasting is like taking a dangerous curve too quickly. Emptiness in the stomach causes dizziness, nausea, and drowsiness. Imagine that you're a tower inhabited by a ravenous beast who is protesting and violently shaking the walls of that tower. It's something like that. Once again, the waiting room was filled with inflated comrades reading women's magazines, but this time with expressions of dread and glucose remorse on their faces. They called us in one by one, first to drink down a disgusting brew that masqueraded as orange juice but with twice the sugar. Then we went back to our corners, mumbling profanities at the nurses, to wait for them to call us into the slaughterhouse again to extract our blood. This procedure would repeat four times over the course of three long hours during which we alternated between ingesting the orange thing and being jabbed with needles. I left there with bruised arms. And on top of everything, I'd have to wait an eternal week for the results.

I couldn't continue the job with the veterinary association because just the thought of walking up that hill from the metro station to the office every day with my now quite considerable belly made my hair stand on end. Maybe I could still have managed it at that point, but at eight or nine months it sounded diabolical. I kept expanding and my physical capabilities kept shrinking bit by bit. If, at seven months, it was now impossible to climb a small hill without inducing Braxton Hicks contractions that made me feel like I was going into labor, how would I be able to get up for work every day when the due date was even closer?

I had as reference some women I'd seen working while very pregnant. In Lima, for example, I remembered the typical pregnant woman begging at stoplights. From Barcelona, I remembered a girl in my old office who had worked up until the seventh month and then had gone to her gynecologist and asked him to sign a "high risk" maternity leave form, which is like disability leave. So she stopped working at seven months but still continued to receive seventy-five percent of her salary. Although this kind of leave is intended for pregnant women who work driving motorcycles, for example, or as city trash collectors, many women resort to this little ruse—maybe because they suffer from water retention, back pain, or another of the usual ailments—and so avoid the difficult situation of having to work all the way up until the end of their pregnancies.

While all of my pregnant sisters past their seventh month were looking for ways to get out of their jobs, I, paradoxically, was looking to get into one. Don't try to understand it. I just had to. My future depended on it. So I called a friend who worked for a publisher who had given me some small assignments during my first months in Barcelona. Only a friend would hire a woman who's seven months pregnant and planning to take occupational risk leave at the first sign of trouble. I explained the entire problem to him and, in two minutes, the publisher had given me a limited-term contract. Enough time to get my affairs in order.

I began going in to the office, once again to enter names into a database, but this time it was people's names rather than dogs'. The novel part was accepting that I was a charity case, which produced in me feelings of both gratitude and shame. Despite everything, I tried to carry it off with dignity, responding with extreme friendliness to all of the secretaries' questions about my "serious" condition and allowing them to spoil me just because I was going to be a mother and didn't have a pot to piss in. I had renewed belief in the power of pregnant women to attain anything they set their minds to.

I went back to the hospital the following week. I fingered the envelope the receptionist had just handed to me and I walked over to the window where there was better light. I felt like throwing up, but I contained myself. I opened it. There was the word I'd dreamed of finding: negative. I did not have diabetes. I let out a sigh of relief. That night I celebrated with a few churros with *dulce de leche*. The next day, I went to see Eulalia who, after performing a general physical exam, concluded that I had too much fat around my middle and that I should watch my weight in any case, cut my adored *Cacaolat* chocolate milk from my diet, and eat more peeled fruit and boiled vegetables, thus avoiding toxoplasmosis while I was at it.

Toxoplasmosis is one of the bogeymen of pregnancy because it can seriously affect the fetus. It's an infectious disease caused by parasites (carried by cats, birds, and other domestic animals) that is transmitted to humans through contaminated food or undercooked meat. I started to feel frightened and I asked Eulalia what I could do to be sure that my baby was fine, since the ultrasounds were done so far apart. Maybe I could come into the doctor's office to listen to her heartbeat every time I felt worried?

"You have to pay attention," Eulalia said. "If you notice that she hasn't moved in a while, you should lie down and see if you can feel her moving. If not, you can eat something to activate her."

Activate her? So the little critter could simply deactivate like a battery-powered rabbit? She'd insisted from the beginning on her determination to be born and now she was depending on me to charge her batteries?

My diet, much to my chagrin, had to grow more disciplined in the wake of the false alarm with the diabetes. By the end of my seventh month, I was eating bread with ham and cheese for breakfast, a yogurt mid-morning, fruit all day long (especially grapefruit, which I'd become addicted to), a robust and variable lunch based on pasta or lentils or garbanzos or rice with peppers and mushrooms or a potato and spinach puree, grilled meat, fish, chicken, or shrimp; and always an enormous salad with cucumbers, cabbage, carrots, radishes, tomatoes, and lettuce. At night, just a sandwich and a glass of milk. Sometimes I said to hell with the diet and ate chicken nuggets from McDonald's, pizza, or a lemon sorbet.

And so, at my last visit with Eulalia, I had lost two pounds. That day, in addition to weighing me, the midwife gave me a piece of good news: Magdalena-Lena was head down, she had rotated, and the pressure I was feeling in my ribs was thanks to her transparent feet. She was in position. The next week I would begin my birthing classes.

That afternoon, I got an email response from Irene, the esteemed La Leche League member I'd seen in Lima and who, in recent days, had become my trusty advisor via phone and email. Irene would analyze and comment on every change I experienced, while I tried to take maximum advantage of her still-fresh knowledge about pregnancy, lactation, and child-rearing. In her last message, she'd expressed her happiness that I didn't have diabetes, especially because, she said, the children of diabetic mothers had to have their blood drawn frequently in order to control their sugar levels. In the hospital, her roommate's poor little baby's legs had been covered in red prick marks. As for me, though I had escaped diabetes, I continued to struggle with sciatica. The four hours I worked sitting down in the office, plus those I spent writing at home, just about unhinged me. Particularly painful was what Eulalia called my pelvic floor. To put it plainly: my ass hurt brutally. It seemed kind of of absurd for my ass to hurt. I called Irene that night, thinking she'd have some sort of answer for me.

"Sorry, Wiener, but I've never heard that one before. When it comes to asses, all I know about are hemorrhoids."

"Well, now that you mention it, that hasn't happened to me yet . . . "

"But it's not a pointless pain. It's just your body preparing itself."

"Okay, okay."

"Did you buy the book?"

"What book?"

"The one I've been recommending to you for weeks. *Kiss Me!* by Carlos González."

"Oh, right. I still need to buy it."

"He has another one called *My Child Won't Eat*, and it's good too, but the other one is amazing. I'm reading another book right now that's also amazing. It's called *The Continuum Concept*. You have to get it."

While pregnancy manuals might have seemed stupid to me, books on how to raise your kids might as well have been written in Sanskrit. Irene didn't know that those books were simply foreign literature, written not for me but for other women who were . . . mothers? I understood that this indifference had nothing to do with the quality or usefulness of the books, but rather with my inability to see myself as a mother. I may, despite myself, have achieved a certain measure of identification with the pregnant women in those online forums or seen myself reflected in those month-by-month fetal chronicles, but I didn't feel like a mom and, what's worse, I had no idea how to go about changing that.

"The continuum concept" alludes to the continuum that should exist for the baby between being inside and outside the mother's body. The way to achieve this is to make sure the baby experiences the transition "in arms." Babies whose continuum needs have been met from the very start develop strong self-esteem and are more independent than babies who, for fear of "spoiling them" or making them too dependent, have been left to cry it out. These needs are: constant physical contact with the mother, sleeping in bed with the parents (co-sleeping) until the baby decides otherwise, breastfeeding on demand, and being carried or strapped to the mother's body until eight months old. This theory of attachment parenting which, I later learned, was embodied by Carlos González, pediatrician and president of the Pro-Breastfeeding Association of Barcelona, was the polar opposite of the controversial routine-based method promoted by Estivill, a doctor specializing in sleep disorders who champions the benefits of allowing babies to cry it out in order to teach them to sleep. No doubt about it, that was not my battle . . . for the moment.

I called my mother to find out which method she had used with me. As always when I try to find out something about my childhood, she got defensive. My mom thinks I try to blame her for all my adult ills, but that isn't completely true. She, too, was once a first-time mother and I'm sure she felt helpless in the face of the avalanche of contradictory information. There was probably a time when she defended her point of view about my upbringing and seized on everything that the science, psychology, and medicine of the 1970s had to offer her as a modern, rationalist, and liberated woman, in order to counteract the home remedies proffered by her own mother. How could I judge her for having let me cry when she believed she was doing the right thing? The truth is that there are some nights, almost always after a fight with J, when I can't sleep without being properly consoled, and if J doesn't feel like making up, I can spend hours crying without stopping until he finally takes me in his arms, and only then do I sleep like a baby. The Estivill method?

In *Perfect Madness*, the *New York Times* columnist Judith Warner criticizes the model of "total motherhood," an intensive approach to mothering that begins with "attachment parenting" and ends with the mother frenetically baking cookies at midnight, attending daily parent meetings and planning a schedule of after-school activities as if the child were the prime minister. In this brand of self-imposed "immersion" motherhood, which Warner describes after having conducted hundreds of interviews with North American women in their thirties, the women have almost no sex and they can't sleep and they have the feeling that they are always doing something wrong. These are women who were raised by feminist mothers who taught them that they could do everything, but who now live in a constant state of angst as they try to single-handedly juggle their responsibilities as professionals, wives, and mothers. For Warner, not only does this represent a second or even third shift, but it is also a genuine disorder that drives many women into tranquilizer addiction.

I called Irene. She was one of those full-time mothers. I asked her if she felt anxious.

"At first I felt lost, stressed, and guilty."

"Because you were sleeping with him?"

"Yes, I told myself it would only be for the first week, then just three months until that tooth came through . . . "

"And then?"

"I felt guilty for always holding him, for not letting him cry. I also felt guilty that I wasn't working or because I didn't take him to a daycare so he could learn to socialize."

"And when did you stop feeling like that?"

"When I listened to my heart. I relaxed and allowed myself to do what I felt was right with total freedom. Finally, my instinct and I got in sync and I am just loving it."

Irene felt stressed out by what society expected of her as a mother, but once she freed herself of external demands she also freed herself of stress. She was surprised that in a country like France, where there was so much social assistance, women detached themselves from their children when they were barely three months old, leaving them in daycare and going back to work in order to maintain their high standards of living.

I wrote to Violeta. She agreed that, for the first time in history, motherhood was being perceived in a joyful way.

"Well, it's a very powerful experience and really demanding, but I think it can be fucking great if you give yourself over to it," she wrote to me. "Of course, this is very difficult for the women of today, because we're living in such competitive times that we're afraid of bullshit like being able to get back into the working world after taking time off, etc. I think we go back and forth between these two forces, and naturally, the one that wins out is the one that most nourishes us, and so motherhood could also become a real nightmare. For me, I feel like it's an experience where the more he gets out of it, the more I get out of it too. His happiness is attuned to my state of mind."

Maybe it was too soon to say, but I did not plan, under any circumstances, to stop working in order to dedicate myself exclusively to my home and my family, and not only because we weren't rich and didn't live off a trust fund, but because I have always enjoyed carrying out my own "personal affairs." Would I be a good mother only if

I renounced what, up until now, I had considered life's pleasures, or would motherhood reveal to me other kinds of pleasures?

With her red high heels and bare legs, Eulalia came into the room packed with women and ceremoniously introduced herself as the leader of our birth preparation course, also know as the Lamaze Method. The first thing she did was ask us to move the chairs into a circle so that she could see all our faces.

"Welcome, everyone. In this course, you will learn a bit more about your process, about how to relax and prepare yourselves for the birth."

The midwife then asked us to pair up with the couple sitting next to us, to tell each other a little about our lives and something about the baby we were expecting, if it was a girl or a boy, the due date, the hospital where we'd be giving birth (I'd be at Barcelona Maternity), and also, if we wanted, we could share a concern or an experience. Then we were supposed to introduce the other couple to everyone else.

Since it was the first day of class, I had dragged J there, thinking about all the times I'd seen those bucolic images of couples preparing themselves for the birth. Luckily, J got off work at the magazine at two o'clock, so he had the whole afternoon free. He would have spent that time watching, for the umpteenth time, one of those movies he loves to watch over and over, but instead, there he was, at my side, looking at me with a "I'm going to kill you and your baby" expression on his face. The truth is that I couldn't have tolerated being in that situation alone, surrounded by the rest of those happy little fat ladies and their husbands.

The round of introductions began. There was one woman about forty years old who said she was a smoker. She was very thin and her belly was really small for being in her eighth month. One couple, a Brazilian dancer and her Catalan husband, who looked like they didn't have a care in the world, were introduced by another couple, a Spaniard and an Ecuadorian woman who was having tremendous back pain. I introduced an older and somewhat overweight couple. The woman's legs were very swollen because of water retention and she was wearing flip-flops that revealed her bloated feet. I told everyone that this was her first baby and that it was a boy.

Suddenly, I realized that I was the only one expecting a girl. The couple next to me introduced me as a journalist whose ass, just at the moment, was really hurting. Eulalia interrupted to ask us to find a mat and to sit in the lotus position, the "dads" hugging the "moms'" bellies from behind. How did these women find it relaxing to sit on the floor? Obviously, I was the only one experiencing ass pain. Eulalia turned off the lights and put on a CD of lullabies. In her nasal voice, she told us how to breathe and what to imagine: she wanted us to think, for example, of a seascape, and to relax in order to connect with our babies. I closed my eyes.

I went to Lamaze classes once a week. On one of those Thursdays, Eulalia greeted us with a gift. It was a supply kit made up of small samples that companies give out to new mothers and future clients. The box was filled with formula and included a bottle and a pacifier. When I told Irene (I knew she'd love hearing that anecdote), she wrote to me in astonishment: "So they give you formula in the hospital before you've even given birth!? Unbelievable." She told me to contact the La Leche League of Barcelona right away and she impressed upon me the importance of learning about breastfeeding, since she herself had paid the consequences of learning only about pregnancy and birth and nothing about nursing. Soon enough, her nipples had cracked, to the point that her baby was drinking milk laced with blood, and she even suffered a breast infection. More horror.

—

GABRIELA WIENER

I think it was the third class that Eulalia dedicated to a discussion of how to prepare the perineum. The perineum is the anatomical part that includes the muscles and skin located in the space between the anus and the vagina, and it's where episiotomies are usually performed, those incisions that allow the baby to come out more easily and which, though not obligatory in Spain, were still performed in ninety-nine percent of cases. A perineum that's in good shape, toned and flexible, Eulalia said as if talking about an arm, will not need an episiotomy or will more easily recover from one.

I've already said that this topic tended to give me night-mares, so I took out a pencil and paper to take notes. Eulalia recommended that that "dads," as she called our husbands, should be in charge of massaging our perinea with some sort of natural oil before going to bed at night.

"This is how we moisturize the perineum," Eulalia elaborated. "Massage in a circular motion to increase circulation and sensitivity in the area."

I don't know if Eulalia knew what she was inciting, but all of the women were smiling and all of the men were looking at each other out of the corners of their eyes.

"When the skin has absorbed all of the oil or lotion, you need to insert your thumb into the vagina and pull gently out and down. Then slide your finger around the walls of the vagina in a 'U' motion, mimicking the sensation of the baby's head as it puts pressure on the perineum."

She also recommended that, at least three times a day, whether in the office, riding the metro, or washing the dishes, we should contract and relax the muscles of the perineum in order to bring more awareness to the space it occupies in our bodies.

"All together now," Eulalia said suddenly, pointing in a graphic manner to her vagina.

"We're going to contract, relax, contract, relax, contract. . . . Very good, just like that, you're doing very well. Keep breathing."

That's how I participated for the very first time in a communal, synchronized perineal exercise session. We all sat there on our mats, imperceptibly contracting our pussies, looking at each other in disbelief as we performed the weirdest aerobics I've ever done in my life.

8

JULY

Baby birds stretch out their necks to ask for food in the presence of their mother, but also in the presence of a long branch whose shadow looks like her.

MARÍA MORENO

FOR THE MAJORITY of animals, breeding stimulates a series of physiological and hormonal mechanisms that cause, in many cases, very odd behavioral patterns. In general, once paired off, couples find themselves driven instinctively to choose a place to settle down and to begin collecting materials with which to build their nests. Every species builds the nest that suits them best. The condor, for example, builds its nest on cliffs in the deep shadows of weathered rocks. I read in the magazine *Cáñamo* that the female goldfinch builds her nest in the most inaccessible branches, on the roofs of buildings, in belfries, in chimneys, on the tops of power poles, and even inside marijuana plants, weaving together roots, stalks, moss, and lichen and lining it with thistledown. When babies are on the way, almost anywhere is a good place to take up residence.

The "nesting instinct" seized me at thirty-one weeks. This pseudo-clinical symptom that affects pregnant women in the third trimester manifests itself as an unstoppable instinct to sweep, wash, iron, and organize everything in our paths, like in a male chauvinist fantasy. In an act of kinship with the animal kingdom, the pregnant woman begins to nest, be it from a case of ribonucleic *déjà vu* or a Pavlovian response to bunny-rabbit wallpaper. The majority of women who have been pregnant report experiencing the nesting urge and it's seen as a race against the clock of prepartum anxiety. Preparing the space where the baby will be, along with the clothes and other things it will need in the first days of life—in short, having everything under control—becomes the impending mother's reason to exist. Even the most slovenly and lazy women become dedicated housewives and, no matter how voluminous they may be, one day you'll find them atop a ladder, cleaning spiderwebs from chandeliers with a feather duster, polishing the hardwood floors at three in the morning or knitting horrible seafoam-green sweaters for a baby who'll be born in the middle of summer. This is all twice as impressive when you consider that an eight-and-a-half-month pregnant woman is a seal, so fat that she can't pluck her own pubic hairs, or verify that she's put on two matching shoes, or pick anything up that's fallen to the floor, and that includes her other child, if she has one. People give us their seats on the metro and the bus, they let us go right to the window at the bank and we even cast our votes during elections without having to stand in line. Everyone seems so concerned about us, asking if it's a boy or a girl, and how much longer until the big event. It's like being famous. There's no privacy whatsoever for a pregnant woman. Now I know how obese women feel, with everyone staring at them all the time. Seriously, it's an exhausting time. And then, right at that particular moment, your hormones tell you to get to work.

A month before the due date I still had absolutely nothing ready. I hadn't organized or cleaned, much less decorated. Apparently, I was supposed to have already packed my suitcase for the hospital, but we hadn't even opened the one we'd stuffed, back in Lima, with size zero unisex baby clothes. It sat behind the door like luggage for a trip that never happened. Everything that people had given to me was lying in a dormant state, stuffed into a bag. Why had I put off this climactic moment, why had I renounced the role I had dreamed of playing one day? Why wasn't I painting little monkeys and clouds on the walls?

I was living in a hundred-square-foot apartment, with two small areas—the bedroom and the living room—separated by a wooden door, a tiny closet-room, a kitchen that could only fit one person at a time, and a bathroom. Ancient wooden window frames let in drafts that tortured us in the winter, along with tons of dust that accumulated on all the furniture. The apartment was adjacent to an abandoned several-story building and, from our enviable rooftop, not only could we see a sliver of the Sagrada Familia, but we also had an exceptional view of the hundreds of pigeons that lived in the empty floors of that building. They were squatter pigeons. The pigeon thing had always been a bizarre feature of our home, and a friend into video art had even come over one day to film them, especially the skylight that they'd converted into their spine-chilling official cemetery, filled not only with fossilized cadavers, but also with various agonizing birds awaiting death. But, for anyone with the smallest sense of sanitation, the pigeons, with their streams of shit, their low-flying flapping and their wide-open common grave, were nothing if not a hub for infections and potential toxoplasmosis. What had been our charming "love nest" during our first years in Barcelona, the envy of so many friends—couples still living with roommates—had now become, courtesy of my nesting instinct, an "old, damp, malignant, reeking rathole in which no child of mine will ever live."

But moving in this city is as complicated as emigrating from one country to another. A house is like El Dorado. For what you pay in Barcelona for a single room, you could be enjoying an entire apartment in a residential neighborhood in Lima, and for what you pay for a mediocre flat, you could have a luxurious ocean-front penthouse. The requirements are a bureaucratic nightmare, and if you happen to be an immigrant to boot, they're a subterranean form of discrimination: collateral, bank guarantees, astronomical deposits. If it's hard for a Spaniard, for foreigners like us it's beyond epic. I tried to come around to the idea that we could revamp our little apartment, clean the dust and paint it from top to bottom, somehow board up access to the pigeon house, throw away all the furniture we'd taken from dumpsters and buy new furniture, renovate the windows, convert the small closet room into a nursery for the baby, but the list grew longer and longer and on into infinity, right along with my anxiety. Could the nesting instinct be fatal?

Both things, staying or leaving, would require enormous amounts of energy, enormous amounts of money, and enormous amounts of time. Everything we lacked.

Were we going to let the pigeons, those flying rats, go on living better than we did?

Third and final appointment with the Spanish Public Health Service, all expenses covered, for which one must be grateful, despite its downsides. This was one of the most important appointments because I would be registering for the first time at Barcelona Maternity, the hospital where Lena would be born. In order to do this, I had to be seen by one of the center's midwives. I was greeted by a Latin American-looking nurse, who I later found out was Bolivian, though she spoke some Catalan. It made me happy to know that I'd be attended to by an almost-compatriot. I would have liked to be able to speak well of her, but that's not the case. She was short and plump, with cropped black hair, and her white coat was too big for her. She took out my clinical history and began reviewing it, asking also for my previous ultrasounds. She started by asking if I smoked, how many cigarettes, if I'd ever taken drugs, if I drank. Generally speaking, I like talking about my past and I always tend to narrate it as fully as I can without sparing any details, especially when it comes to the days when I was using drugs. Suddenly, when I was right in the middle of my story, there was a knock on the door. Two men with the construction crew working on remodels to that floor of the hospital interrupted the appointment to ask if they could take a look at that exam room. She let them come in and go about their work, which seemed unnecessary to me since we were in the middle of my appointment, in the middle of something, something that concerned either my baby or my criminal record. The men brought in a ladder and started to poke at something in the ceiling. Suddenly, a section of paint and concrete came loose and fell to the floor, sprinkling the exam table and everything around it with dust. The workers left and that's when the midwife invited me to lie back on the table so she could examine me. I looked at the disaster the men had left behind and declined to lie down. I told her I was sorry, but I wasn't going to get naked in the middle of that disaster area.

"Of course, of course, whatever you want . . . " she said, adding: "If only our hospitals 'over there' were like this, and all they had was a little dust."

Apparently, this midwife was not pleased with me and had decided to give me a lecture on humility by reminding me of our common and dusty origins. I nodded. I didn't deal well with conflict, be it because of my pregnant-woman's hypersensitivity or my habitual passivity and complicity in the face of aggression, the consequence of years of being bullied in grammar school. She went on subjecting me to a frankly police-like interrogation.

"Abortions?"

"What? Doesn't it say in there? Three."

"What methods of birth control did you use?"

"Condoms, mostly."

"Well, you should really think about using a more continual method like the pill, because the majority of pregnancies happen right after having a baby. You think it's safe and . . . "

"No, I really don't want to go on the pill or anything."

"Well, if you end up pregnant you can just take care of it like you usually do . . . " that bitch said to me.

" . . . What do you mean?" I asked her, not fully under-standing or, more accurately, not believing my ears.

"Do you work?"

I was on the verge of tears.

That horrible woman would attend to me during the difficult hours of labor? Those hands would be the first to touch my daughter and they'd be the ones to suction the mucus from her nose? Now I finally understood that Birth is Ours Association manifesto that denounces the lack of obstetrical rigor and presents cases of women who have suffered from substandard care during pregnancy, unnecessary cesareans, or traumatic deliveries. I was familiar with the heartbreaking testimonies of women who had lost their children because of medical decisions and malpractice. Letters like "To Lucía, Up in Heaven," are among the saddest things I've ever read. But not even reading those letters had managed to set off my alarm bells like this woman sitting in front of me, who appeared to think it her duty to reprimand an irresponsible pregnant woman who had used drugs and had abortions and now wore inadequate shoes, not to mention wanting to have a natural birth as if she thought it were child's play.

"I'm a journalist," I answered her finally.

I was fairly used to people in this country looking at me and immediately lumping me in with the thousands of Peruvian women who have come to Spain to clean houses and take care of the elderly. I didn't usually bother to disabuse them of that notion, but this woman had to know the truth, even if, at the moment, it was a lie.

"I'm an investigative journalist and I'm writing a book about the quality of care pregnant mothers receive from the Public Health Service."

A beautiful expression (at least to me) froze on her face.

I walked away from her as fast as I could, certain that one day I would write about her cruelty and about our deceptive helplessness.

We were finally able to borrow enough money to move, but we still faced the hardest part: finding an apartment. I filled a page with phone numbers and spent hours making calls, but it always turned out the same way: just when it seemed that we were close to finding the perfect apartment, something would go awry. Either it was an interior apartment with no light or it was on the fifth floor with no elevator or it was a hovel or was located in the ass end of nowhere. The nesting instinct was oppressing my brain.

I started trying through word of mouth, telling everyone I knew that we were looking for a place. And so it happened that a couple we knew who were going to be working in Russia for a year offered us their four-bedroom, fully furnished apartment. One strike against it was that we'd have to leave after a year and face another critical "relocation moment," except this time with a baby along for the ride. Finally, another friend told me about an apartment for rent in the same building where a friend of hers lived, a friend who happened to be the brother-in-law of the building's owner. Thanks to that, we secured unbeatable move-in terms and conditions.

That afternoon, J and I went to see the apartment, both of us with a hunch that we were at last going to find our home there. We were out of time to keep looking. It was a good building, it had an elevator, the neighborhood was a bit drab but it was very close to Gracia and the Sagrada Familia. The manager showed us the apartment, which was full of things . . . useless things. The woman told us that, up until recently, a little old lady had lived there, but when she left, no one had come to claim the furniture or any of the woman's belongings, so we could do whatever we wanted with them, keep them or, more logically, she said, throw them away.

But we were no more logical than the goldfinch in the marijuana plant. The apartment was five times bigger than our current place. The furniture was from the '50s, almost in its entirety. One of those enormous gold-framed velvet "paintings" depicting a hunting scene with tigers leaping about against a red background presided over the living room. A "Persian" rug spread across the floor from wall to wall. The dining room table was enormous and heavy. An over-the-top classical chandelier hung from the ceiling. The sideboard, which, months later, an artist friend of ours described as "mid-century hideous," also spanned from wall to wall. The master bedroom came complete with a stately bed, another catastrophic chandelier, and a four-door armoire that took up half the room. None of the furniture was a valuable antique, it was simply ugly, solid, and built to last. There was a still-functional television identical to the one my grandmother owned. The stove and the refrigerator worked too. The house-museum was crowned by a collection of hundreds of postcards that had been mailed from all over Spain to Mrs. Pilar and family. The Pradales, which was the family's last name, had rented that house since 1953. The children had left, the husband had died, and the wife had remained there alone. Over time, she started to fall and break bones and was spending more time in the hospital than in the house, so the children decided it would be better if she went to live in a retirement home.

We also found a photo album, cassette tapes with prayers to Jehovah (they were Witnesses), ten Bibles, an extensive library that hadn't been updated since 1975, a button collection, and all manner of other sorts of things that people leave behind. Thanks to these details, we were able to reconstruct in our imaginations the life that had preceded us.

The most important discovery was another suitcase, the third in this story, but this one was full of vintage sunglasses, some of which were huge and extravagant and had never been worn. Apparently, Mr. Pradales had been a door-to-door salesman for a glasses company. We thought immediately of throwing a sunglasses party for our friends. We decided that it was worth it to move solely because of that suitcase.

We ended up with the suitcase, the apartment, and everything inside it.

After all, it's not like we had anything else to fill the place with.

"The standard rituals of preparing for a baby centered on consumer choices," writes Juliet B. Schor in her book *Born to Buy*, a study about the impact of marketing strategies directed at children. Indeed, more and more, like Christmas or Mother's Day, the arrival of a baby is an event mediated by purchases, a joyful moment filled with consumer pleasures, money spent or debt acquired in order to buy that luxury item called "quality of life." While I might be a thrifty immigrant who has been wearing the same coat and the same pair of boots for years, my daughter would have a bedroom every bit as nice as Tom Cruise's daughter, or my name's not Gabriela Wiener.

A pregnant woman is an easy target, little more than a sitting duck. So, just as I allowed myself to be sucked in by the nesting instinct, I also appeared to be an easy mark for baby-related consumption syndrome. Walking down the street, my eyes were drawn to shop windows in which children's rooms straight out of fantasy were recreated. Also, ever since I'd started attending birthing classes, my name had ended up in the databases of every brand making products for babies and my mailbox filled up every day with ads and magazines featuring photos of pregnant-lady fashion victims who used tons of creams and calendar babies whose every need has been met. The idea was to convince me that my baby needed a "physiological bottle," the texture of which "was the closest thing to a mother's breast." Its magical form, of course, "prevented hiccups and colic." It was "the bottle your baby would ask for if he could." Marketing for baby products was not immune to the ecological angle, the idea being that artificial options ought to look as natural as possible: baby carriers made by Bjorn were "just like carrying your baby inside you." Not to mention: "Baby Monitors with DECT technology: you and your baby will maintain continual, stable, and truly private communication; a real connection." And if that weren't enough, there was the Tummy Tub that "reproduces the conditions of the mother's womb." For advertisers, we mothers were like birds who, instead of gathering twigs and bits of fluff for the nest, bought furniture and state-of-the-art, environmentally conscious gadgets.

With ever-increasing visions of baby products swirling through my mind, I remembered what my friend Irene had told me: "Buy yourself a big bed. Period." She, who had certainly not read the part in the Dada Manifesto about "What is useless is indispensable," but rather "What is essential is invisible to the eye," from *The Little Prince*, maintained that we would be sleeping with the baby for a long time and it was essential for the three of us to be comfortable in the bed. That we didn't need anything else. For her, the crib, the supposed nexus of a baby's life, was of secondary importance. She told me that she'd prepared a beautiful room for her son, with everything a proper nursery ought to have, but it had ended up being totally useless except as a storeroom for the toys awaiting their turn to be used. And don't even mention the stroller. Irene said it was necessary to carry the baby strapped to your body with a length of fabric called a *foulard*.

But I, in my consumerist vortex, clung to the popular belief: a baby without a layette is like a bride without a gift registry, like a mother without a bouquet of roses, like a teenage girl without a teddy bear. I love lists and I make tons of them, though in the end I never manage to complete them. My list was as follows: a crib with crib bedding, a standing baby bathtub and changing table with trays for diapers and baby cleansing products, an armoire and a dresser with drawers for baby clothes, a vibrating baby swing, a sterilizer, an infrared baby monitor, curtains, a lamp, a sofa to nurse her on, a pail for dirty diapers, a humidifier, an activity play mat, and a sleep sack. The baby's wardrobe was another matter: pajamas, onesies, jackets, sweaters, dresses, pants, hats, sweatshirts, bibs, towels, socks, booties, and, of course, enough diapers to carpet all of Latin America. For her part, the mother needed about ten different products that, suspiciously, are all related to breastfeeding: beginning with an electric breast pump and moving on to nipple shields, nursing pads, manual extractors, and the list goes on. It seemed obvious that my tits were in trouble.

If the birth of a baby is a ritual of consumption, Ikea is the sacred temple that every future proletarian mother should frequent as a regular devotee. Our move had been easy, a few trips on the metro with boxes of books and suitcases of clothes, though I didn't do any of it this time around and I couldn't paint the walls on my own either. With the help of a few friends, week by week, we painted a new room. We used bold colors: reds and oranges. The most arduous part was getting rid of the most grotesque of the furniture, taking it apart piece by piece to be able to get it through the door. We decided that even though we appreciated kitsch, we didn't need to go overboard: out went the rug, the curtains, the hunting painting, the chandeliers, the marble tables, and the colossal sideboard. We surprised ourselves by choosing the best and brightest bedroom for little Lena, and taking the ugly one with no natural light for ourselves. Was this filial love? We turned the third bedroom into a sun-dappled study. Instead of giving us things, our friends took up a collection and gave us money for us to invest in whatever we liked. That was when we made a beeline straight to Ikea.

I'm always surprised at the number of things that I don't want to do that I end up doing and the number of things that I want to do that I can't do. I had once been branded a "shopping mall communist" for the way in which theory and practice clashed within me. I embraced the hippie ideology out of pure expediency. I chose to inherit more than I bought. First I acquired the big bed Irene had recommended, in which the three of us would sleep for the first few days. Instead of moving the crib into our bedroom, we would move our bed into Lena's room. It was an odd thing to do, but hers was the nicest room in the house and, this way, we could all share it. There was just one small detail: the floor in Lena's room became a target of my obsession because it was cold tile rather than hardwood. At Ikea, we discovered that they sold hardwood flooring by the foot that you could install yourself just by following the instructions. Every afternoon when he got home from work, J would go into Lena's room and spend several hours working on the floor until, at last, it was ready. In the end, I spent almost nothing on furniture: a friend gave me a crib, changing table, and stroller that had belonged to her daughter. That's another truism about pregnancy: the solidarity between mothers and future mothers. That saying about every baby arriving with a loaf of bread under its arm is almost always courtesy of other women. My friend Aixi, for example, had already given me several tons of clothes that her daughter had outgrown, so Lena's wardrobe was covered for the entire first year, which was great since buying clothes was prohibitively expensive. And, to placate Irene, Aixi had also loaned me a *foulard* I could use to strap the baby to my body, like Andean women did with their children. Mother and child, body to body. The continuum. It was all very *à la mode*.

It was also fashionable, though perhaps from the other end of the spectrum, to blog about your baby. A baby without a blog is just like an adult without a blog: a total weirdo. The Internet is also saturated with the diaries of the still in-utero set. The idea is to tell the baby's story from its first days in the mother's womb, a chronicle meant especially for friends and family who can now find out all about the baby's development by simply typing in a URL. Goodbye to individual emails and telephone calls. These apocryphal blogs are narrated in the first person by loving parents who do not hesitate to impersonate their preliterate offspring. "Hi, I'm Erik and my parents love me very much. I'm happy inside my mommy's belly, but soon I'll come out of here and you'll get to meet me. For now, you can see my first photo, or ultrasound, as they call it. Aren't I handsome?" There are all kinds of blogs, some with special sections dedicated to the layette, in which the expectant parents have posted a photographic panorama of the well-appointed nursery, right down to their little one's future socks. Baby blogs have their own links to other baby blogs and these have links to still others, so there are hundreds of parent communities blogging about their babies, posting photos, videos, pictures of their vaccination charts, and photo albums of their milestones, from the first tooth to the first trip to the zoo. These parents share information and post congratulatory comments for one another. Some blogs even have a counter that keeps track of the days the "author" has been alive: "María is 830 days old." These days, the dilemma of when to stop writing a child's blog has come

to be equally or more important than the actual wean-
ing process.

They say that the nesting instinct coincides with the
beginning of maternity leave, when the future mother
can finally leave the rest of her concerns behind and focus
on the central role she must now play. And yes, I would
probably never again have the time to rub cream into
my nipples, to sign up for swimming and yoga classes. I
thought the moment would never come, but after several
failed attempts to arrive at the office with even a little
oxygen left in my lungs, I had to request maternity leave
and stop working. I would finally get to experience what
it felt like to be a woman with all the time in the world
to putter in her garden and bake pies. But it wasn't like
that. The period of disability had begun.

For example, I was on the brink of putting myself on
leave from sex, despite the fact that all the books encourage you to keep having it until shortly before the birth,
even recommending positions to correspond with each
trimester. I even read that a group of Malaysian doctors
conducted a study that concluded that sex during the final
phase of pregnancy led to a better birth. But between the
constant urge to pee, the Braxton Hicks contractions and
my trouble sleeping, I preferred to encourage J to invest

his energy in other things, such as finishing painting the house or hanging shelves. This excited me a whole lot more.

In my last birthing class, Eulalia had the brilliant idea to show us a video of a birth as a type of grand finale. One woman vomited, and almost all of us cried. We were too close to "that."

The next week I went to a lecture on "Natural Birth" at Barcelona Maternity, the hospital where I'd be giving birth. As I've said, it was the only place in all of Spain with a natural birth protocol, which means more or less the following:

1. Not medicalized (no IVs or oxytocin).
2. Your membranes are not artificially ruptured.
3. You are permitted to move around during dilation.
4. You are permitted to deliver in the position of your choice.
5. Forceps and vacuum extraction are not used.
6. Monitoring of the baby is external and sporadic.
7. Analgesics and anesthesia (epidural) are not used.

I will never forget what the midwife leading the discussion with our group of "brave women" who wanted to give birth "in pain" said to us:

"Natural birth. . . . Ha ha ha ha."

The damned woman assured us that we'd end up screaming for an epidural. Her opinions caused general indignation. Also, she didn't fail to warn us that there was only one delivery room outfitted with all the necessities for natural birth. So it would be first come, first served. May the best belly win.

By that point, my level of consciousness and commitment to natural birth was such that I even insulted my sister-in-law for having sought a C-section in a private clinic where they tended to do many more C-sections than in public hospitals since vaginal birth is so much less expensive.

I still hadn't packed my suitcase with the things I'd be taking to the hospital, but there was still time. Technically, I still had two more weeks. Plenty of time to create the baby's Facebook account.

JULY 29TH

Life changes fast.
Life changes in the instant.
You sit down to dinner
and life as you know it ends.

JOAN DIDION

I ONCE MADE a collage in which I fantasized about the physical appearance of a hypothetical child J and I might have. I titled it "Freaks." I cut up photos of each of us and tried out a series of different possible combinations: a boy with J's hair + my eyes + J's nose + my mouth. A girl with my hair + J's eyes + my nose + J's mouth. A child like a puzzle put together at random, a Frankenstein's monster made of chopped-up parts, a Minotaur without a labyrinth. It was like playing God. The vision had frightened me so much (and it wasn't even a collage of our psychological attributes) that I subtitled it: "There are already enough monsters in this world." I made it with the certainty that we were never going to have children.

Years after that graphic declaration of my intentions, I stood before my rounded reflection in the mirror, waiting for the moment in which my life would change forever thanks to the collage that Mother Nature had assembled for us. Every one of these more or less transcendental visions vanished when I caught sight of the stain in my underwear, a kind of dark slime that clung to my fingers as I scrutinized it from a distance of about two centimeters. I'd had sex with J the day before and I thought it was some kind of congealed semen residue. I immediately called Eulalia. Maybe the baby's nose had fallen off.

"It's the mucus plug," the midwife told me, very calm.

"What's that?"

"It's the membrane that protects the cervix and protects the baby from germs."

"Does this mean she's coming? But I still have two weeks!" I screamed hysterically. My need for her to be born was as huge as my fear that it would finally happen and I vacillated, as always, between desire and denial.

"No, it doesn't mean she's coming today, just that the birth is approaching . . ."

"At more or less what speed?"

"Well, it could be tomorrow or anytime in the next two weeks. Oh, and you shouldn't have sex. Without the plug, the fetus is exposed to outside infections, okay?"

Okay. No sex and awash in uncertainty. A fine how-do-you-do.

The day when life as I knew it would begin to change forever, I got up with the idea of going out to buy cold compresses. It was the only thing left on my equipment list that I still needed. Compresses for the bleeding I'd experience immediately postpartum. I headed for the pharmacy. But as I walked, I kept thinking of more things that we needed at the house. I went to the fruit stand and bought some tomatoes and limes; I went to the bakery for bread and to the corner store for a jug of water. I bought a rotisserie chicken. I walked home, stumbling and panting. I had as much energy as a coked-up soccer player but the coordination and agility of a mammoth. I told J over the phone what I'd done. He told me I was crazy. I took a bath. I went into Lena's room to meditate. Recently, I'd been meditating several times a day. I found the melon color of the walls and the recently completed hardwood floors relaxing. I would go in there, make sure that everything was in its place and inhale the air deodorizer, filling my lungs. I would stand by the lonely crib, running my finger along its bars in search of traces of dust. I would think of her as I looked at the baby clothes, hugged a little woolen dog, touched the bristles on the small hairbrush and smelled the diaper rash cream. During those hours, I discovered I was missing something that hadn't happened to me yet, someone I hadn't yet had the pleasure of meeting. I remembered going into my grandmother's bedroom shortly after her death. Every one of her things evoked her, sent me backwards into the past. Here, in an unborn baby's bedroom, it was the opposite: everything projected into the future.

Yet in both places the emptiness took on a shape.

After lunch that afternoon I once again opened the suitcase I'd take to the hospital. A pregnant woman's suitcase is like Sport Billy's Omni-Sack, but encoded in some stupid way. You spend days tinkering with it, like a poem you've just written. You read it and it seems amazing, then you reread it and decide it's a piece of shit. Packing a suitcase for you and your baby can be thrilling: how will you dress it on its first day of life? Another science fiction-worthy topic: What would the baby want to wear on her first day outside my belly? J never let me pick out his clothes, so I felt fulfilled. I chose a light-blue onesie with small flowers, a pair of tiny striped pants and a little blue jacket. I was overcome by diminutives. The package of size zero diapers was ready and waiting in the suitcase, along with the little receiving blanket, the four changes of teensy clothing, including onesies, little pants, pajamas, petite gowns, tiny socks, a miniature hat, a pair of prissy nightgowns for me, my toiletries, a towel, a book and the iPod. Apparently, the idea is to keep yourself entertained with something while you're suffering horrendous pain. Irene had recommended that I take something to eat, since you go hours without food and then, in the end, you won't have the energy to push; deep down I knew that this was one of her subversive pieces of advice, since the hospital usually forbids patients from eating whenever they want to. And all of my books warned me not to eat or drink anything before the birth. Nevertheless, I put a banana, an apple, and a package of crackers in a bag.

After eating, I lay down on the couch to watch TV. It was basically all I was capable of doing. Except more eating, of course. Every time I lay down I'd be beset by painless contractions, though now they didn't see so painless to me. J came home from the office and told me he was going out that night. Something like a last hurrah. He was planning to meet up with a few friends. He started checking his email while we were chatting about our days. I started feeling strange. The pains were like menstrual cramps, but they were growing more and more intense. It was 8:00 p.m. when I signaled red alert.

"I think you should go now," I told J in a manipulatively doleful tone. "And you shouldn't stay out too late. I wouldn't want to go into labor when you're not here and then have you feel like the guiltiest man on the planet."

J looked at me condescendingly.

"I sent them a text an hour ago saying I wasn't going."

I was happy. Every time he stays with me I feel happy. I'm a possessive bitch. I don't have a life of my own. I'm the type of woman who suffers waiting for her man, like the women in José Luis Perales's songs. And now that I have a baby in my belly, I'm scared. I may be other things too, but those aren't really relevant at the moment.

The suitcase. I remembered the suitcase. I'd checked it, but I'd still managed to forget to put in the sanitary pads I'd bought that morning, when I'd squandered so much energy that I suspected I was now going into labor with such shocking swiftness that I was about to give birth right then and there, despite the fact that the due date wasn't until August 12.

"Today is July 28. Peruvian Independence Day!" I shrieked in terror. "What'll we do if she's born today? It's a horrible day to be born. My grandfather was born on July 28 and we always spend his birthday watching the parade and listening to the president's speech. Poor girl."

"And I haven't finished painting yet," said J.

Or gotten rid of all the old furniture. And my parents were supposed to arrive on the eighth.

I looked around: except for Magdalena's room, the house was a half-painted mess. I felt another contraction. When it passed, I ran to put the cold compresses in the suitcase and looked through it one more time to be sure I wasn't forgetting anything. That was the last gesture of forethought I would be allowed. After that moment, everything would be a constant chain of unfolding outcomes.

So these were the fucking contractions. Or should I call them contradictions? Abdominal pain like during your period and lower back pain like a kidney stone. With every contraction, the belly gets so hard it seems like it will explode. I wouldn't be able to endure much of this. It was 11:00 p.m. I cried in J's arms, terrified.

"Okay, calm down," he said, stroking my hair. "We have to wait for them to be more regular."

I felt like the first time I took Ayahuasca. What was the use of all my incredulity, my cynicism, if I would now have to surrender to the evidence? It was all true. The fear, the pain, one's own truth. It was a transporting experience. That's why it's called a delivery.

J had been glued to his watch for a while now and was recording the frequency of my contractions. I'd been suffering lashing pains that reverberated through my back and belly for at least two hours. I was wobbling from one end of the house to the other. When a contraction hit, I would grab onto J as though bombs were falling on our heads. Despite the pain, I managed one last civic effort and whipped up a colon cleanse, like a porno actress preparing, with great dignity, for a double penetration. There we were, J and I, like so many couples who'd attended birthing classes, who've read infinite self-help books, there we were and we had no fucking idea what to do.

The pain had me crying out for my mother. I only call for my mom when something hurts me a lot, physically or emotionally. What were we doing alone in this country without our moms? Reckless fucking idiots! And why weren't they here? Suddenly, the stark reality hit me:

"They're going to miss the birth!"

My parents were coming but they'd bought their tickets for August 8. I called my mother to give her the bad news.

"My poor girl, everything is going to be okay," she told me, trying to share in my desperation. Her voice broke as she told me that she was imagining she was giving me massages. Her voice only made me cry harder. I needed her.

They say that the way in which a woman handles labor pain is more or less the way she handles everything else in life, including death. I wasn't exactly coming out smelling like roses.

I talked to my dad and then to my sister. Everyone was nervous. They wished me luck as if I were going away on a trip. Conclusion: I could die. I talked to my mother-in-law, to my brother-in-law. On the verge of asphyxiation, I said goodbye to all of them in my mind, like that time when I got swamped by a wave at the beach in La Punta and I saw my life flash before me like in a movie. And right at that moment, another contraction almost killed me. We hung up. We had to go to the hospital, even at the risk of looking ridiculous if they sent us right back home. I didn't care how many times I'd heard the story of the woman who goes to the hospital too early. We called a taxi to take us as soon as possible to someplace where they'd know what to do with me.

En route to Barcelona Maternity. At midnight I heaved a sigh of relief: my daughter had been spared being born on the same day as Alberto Fujimori, the ex-president of Peru. On the other hand, the taxi driver was a total asshole, like almost all taxi drivers in this city. He was worried that I would stain his upholstery. The good part was that, for this same reason, he drove like a bat out of hell and we got there in a flash.

When we arrived, they took us to Emergency. It was full of pregnant women and their overly attentive husbands. The majority of them had come in on a false alarm and were now hooked up to one of those monitors that measures the frequency of contractions. One pregnant lady was smoking. They took note of my contrite expression and asked me to take off my underwear and lie down on a stretcher. By this point I could barely do anything for myself. In the neighboring stretcher lay another woman with a titanic belly. We looked at each other and smiled in camaraderie and with a certain equanimity that was quite commendable given our condition. The woman was two weeks overdue. Her face was desperation itself. She was not enjoying herself. She was having a boy, a dilly-dallying boy. I was telling her that I was having a girl when someone abruptly closed the curtain between us. The perpetrator of this elegant gesture was a gaunt woman in a white coat, with black hair tied back in a ponytail, who looked like this wasn't her day or even her year. She didn't even say hello. She opened my legs without a word and put her fingers inside me, an expression of disgust on her face. She didn't like what she saw one bit. She growled, her brow furrowed.

"You're not even three centimeters dilated. Go back home, okay? You still have a long way to go."

"Excuse me, but it's just that this is my first time . . ."

Why was it my destiny to always be attended by people probably being forced to work overtime? This lady had the face of a McDonald's cashier at 11:00 p.m. Okay, it's a tough job, but. . . . On the day advertised as "the happiest day of my life," was I going to have to put up with that woman's sneer just because I couldn't afford a private clinic? I'd already been warned that it was the luck of the draw and I might end up with the "cranky" midwife. I told her I was in a lot of pain and asked her to move me into a hospital room where I might feel more at ease as I continued dilating and waited for the big moment to arrive.

"Well, what kind of birth are you having?"

"Natural . . ."

"Ugggggg. That can take days. Can't you see what we're dealing with around here? There's no room for you."

"But I don't have a car. Really, I'd prefer to stay. There are no taxis and, anyway, they're not exactly cheap at this hour."

"You can go walk circles around the hospital until your time comes. Come back when your contractions are closer together, okay?"

This said, she left just as she'd arrived. I couldn't even fathom jogging around the hospital in the middle of the night while suffering labor pains. Just as I was getting dressed, two girls came in.

"Hi, how's it going?"

It was two excessively young women, probably interns. Their faces were deceptively angelic.

"Can I examine you down there?" one of them said.

Much later, I remembered that Irene had warned me about "reconnaissance tactics." "Doctors will put their hands inside you to rupture your membranes before you even realize what they're doing," she'd said suspiciously. But in that moment I was defenseless and at the mercy of medical authority, even if that authority was practically prepubescent.

"I guess so . . . "

"It'll just take a minute."

Both girls put on gloves and took up posts in front of my wide-open vagina as if it were a coffee machine. First, one inserted her finger deep inside me. She whispered something to the other girl. Then the second girl did the same. They took off their gloves and tossed them in the trash. They had learned something new for the day.

"Thank you very much."

"Is everything okay?" I asked, to say something.

"Yes, yes, everything's fine."

They left and I had an enormous contraction. They'd used us like guinea pigs. I got dressed as best I could and went to look for J, who was smoking outside like in a birth scene from a movie. When I'd dreamed about the birth, J was in every scene, but so far he was an outcast from his own paternity, a father of the old guard.

Another taxi incident. Outside the hospital, on the corner in front of the Reina Sofía Hotel, another taxi driver fled when he saw that I was pregnant. Incredible. It couldn't be true. We shouted insults. Thank goodness one driver took pity on us. He talked and talked about how awful some drivers are, as if he were discussing the result of a Barça–Recreativo match. I was no longer listening to anything external. It was much better that way.

My natural birth began with an ambulance.

But first we filled the tub with warm water. I undressed and got in. We lit aromatic candles and turned off the light. A bit of mellow music. But it was too late for me to turn into a hippie. So many years of bitterness can't be erased just like that. I lasted ten minutes in the tub and spent the rest of the time dragging myself across the floor. From the bed to the couch and from the couch to the floor. J tried to give me some of those special massages, but it just made me want to hit him.

I'm not going to lie: I was not acting very brave.

I'll have to tell Lena that the day of her birth was the day of the taxis. At six in the morning it was still completely dark. At that particular moment I no longer cared if some cranky nurse thought I wasn't ripe for the plucking. I was completely overcome. I expelled some liquid. It must have been my water breaking. They told me that if the liquid was clear I could still take my time, but if it was dark it meant the baby had pooped inside me and now ran the risk of asphyxiation. In that case we had to come in right away.

The liquid was clear, but I was still ready to hightail it. J called a taxi. They told him there were none available. He called another number and was told the same thing. He got out the phone book and dialed dozens of taxi companies, all with the same result. Some of them told him it could be more than an hour. J explained that it was an urgent situation, that they should drop everything and come get his wife who was about to give birth. I brooded over my misery from a corner of the room. In those days, stingy taxi drivers didn't work on the weekends (now they do, and they charge double). Too many drunks ready to vomit their guts out.

"Why don't we have a car?! Why didn't we ask some-one to drive us?! Why don't we have more friends with cars?!"

Faced with this transportation crisis, any shred of dark humor I might have had left had been replaced by pure desperation.

"Call an ambulance," I begged J.

"Do ambulances come for pregnant women?"

"Tell them it's half out of me, that you can see the head. That there's not one fucking taxi in the entire city."

What a way to kick off my much-heralded natural birth. The ambulance was on the way. They rang the bell in under five minutes. I walked out the door on my own two legs. I did not have to overact. I looked pretty destroyed. The ambulance guys hoisted me into the back. J got in up front. One of those little Emergency Medical Service chicks was waiting for me in the back. I looked at her distrustfully. By that point I was sure that every woman I came across wanted to put her finger inside me. And it was true. She did it. The other technician asked her if I was fully dilated. "The head's in position," she replied. Finally, some good news. And seeing Barcelona from the back of an ambulance also made me feel better. Pure exhibitionism: the sirens and the people turning around to look, imagining someone inside on the brink of death.

It was almost as good as seeing a funeral procession pass by. I felt like Doctor Hannibal Lecter, faking injury and just dying to eat the nurse's nose right off his face.

I arrived at Barcelona Maternity in grand style. That is to say, surrounded by the sirens and red lights of an ambulance. I went in through the back door and made a dramatic entrance into the Emergency Department. My reception was slightly less chilly than it had been the first time around. They opened the doors for us as we approached. Finally, I wasn't an imaginary invalid. I was making up for all the times I'd gone pointlessly to the hospital certain of looming catastrophe (hangovers I'd confused with the onset of a heart attack). Once again, J was stopped at the door and blocked from entering. They determined that I'd only dilated one more centimeter. From two to three. The bearer of this new bad news: the nasty midwife. Who else? Eulalia would not be there. As I've said, I'd only seen the gynecologist once in my life. The entire time, I was hearing female voices in my head urging me to defend my natural birth with my life. On the other side, I heard the voice of a little devil whispering to me that I should ask for an epidural and be done with it. I took advantage while the noxious midwife was momentarily distracted to ask another of the midwives if that woman was going to be at my birth, because if she was, not only did I want an epidural, but also general anesthesia or even a lethal overdose. The mere possibility of staying there and going through the blessed work of labor, without J, surrounded by these stressed-out people, made me tremble.

"No, in a little while they'll move you upstairs. Don't worry," she told me with a wink.

"Natural birth?"

"Yes."

"Good."

Good? The contractions had taken the form of thousands of missiles embedding themselves in my midsection.

With any luck, in a few hours I was going to have one less enemy in the world.

I won't belabor the story too much.

Belabor: the irony of the word hurts.

I arrived in a wheelchair to the "Dilation" area. That's where everything starts to seem like one of those tear-jerker hospital TV shows. And me, hallucinating that House would appear from behind the curtains, ready to rupture my membranes with his cane.

The staff on this floor was noticeably different from the Emergency Department staff. But they didn't look like House. I was received by a stocky gay nurse who was cheerful in a way that, in any other circumstance, could have been called "contagious."

"I know it hurts, sweetie, just hang in there."

In the blink of an eye I had traded the witch for a teddy bear. Before me appeared the room of my dreams. The much-sought-after natural birth room was mine, all mine: a single room, with a view of the clinic's interior courtyard, a bathroom with a bathtub, a birthing chair, a gigantic ball and, the most important thing of all: J and I in complete privacy, technology at the service of nature. I'd take it.

"What are you going to name your baby girl?"

If the nurse starts chatting it's a very bad sign. It means you're about to suffer murderous pain.

"Magdalena."

"What?! What do you mean you're going to name her Magdalena? Today is Saint Marta's day! She's Magdalena's sister, for God's sake! You have to name her Marta! Magdalena's day was July 22. You already missed it, sister! Hahahaha. You have to name her Marta! Marta!"

I could scarcely respond. I didn't have even half of his conviction, basically in any aspect of my life.

"I don't like the name Marta. It's totally boring."

This was surreal. This saint's day aficionado nurse was telling us that were about to give our daughter the wrong name. Marta is the dutiful sister, the one who complains about everything, the one who compares herself to others and goes to tell Jesus that Magdalena is an unreliable such and such who loafs about all day long and leaves all the work for her to do. Nevertheless, Jesus chooses Magdalena, the weepy slut, as a model of the contemplative soul, and he questions Marta's agitation. The odd thing is that Marta, the little snitch, is the saint, the patron saint of innkeepers, and not Magdalena. Like I would ever name my baby Marta!

"Well, guys, you've arrived just at our shift change."

"No!!" I screamed. "Don't leave us! We'll name her Marta!"

And now who would come? He was leaving just as I was beginning to feel some iota of human warmth.

"Don't worry, everything will be fine."

We were alone. And I couldn't bear to lie down. I started walking in circles around the room, crying and calling out for my mom again. I went into the bathroom. I sat in the bathtub. J gave me a massage. I sat on the ball and bounced up and down. For the first time, I started to think that I couldn't handle it. Shit, the truth is that for a couple of hours now I hadn't thought of anything else except getting the epidural and putting an end to all this. I cursed every one of the sinister midwives.

"Good morning, how are you?" A short, young woman came into the room. "My name's Raquel. What's your name?"

"Gabriela."

"And the baby?"

"It's a girl. Her name's Magdalena."

"What a pretty name."

Well, that was something at least. This midwife seemed like my cup of tea. She was very sweet and it was clear she wanted to convey a sense of tranquility. She told me that she usually attended home births, that she followed in the footsteps of the ancient doulas, the women who, for millennia, have helped other women to give birth. She was exactly what I needed.

I saw the light.

"Now then," she said, deeply massaging my back and hips, her voice almost hypnotic. "The contractions are like waves, you see? They come and go, they pass through your body. Feel how they pass through and then they go away. Feel how the pain passes through you and then releases you. Allow it to flow through you. Don't flee from it, feel it fully. Concentrate on it, let it open you like a flower, look inside yourself."

I half lay down on the bed, my feet still on the floor. I liked that position. Then I got down on all fours. That gave me some relief too. I was feeling much better. I was connecting with my inner self. This mantra thing was working. I looked at J and told him that I could do this.

But the midwife had to go. She was attending to ten other women just like me. I sank right back into my child-ish relationship with the pain. J did his best, but it wasn't the same. I realized I needed that woman to guide me through this. If she had stayed with me, maybe I wouldn't have had to bare my fangs and ask for the epidural.

I was five centimeters dilated and you have to make it to ten, which is when the cervix is completely open and effaced. No drugs work. Not Entonox, a pain-relieving gas, or any of the opiates that I've heard some women use during home births. It was an epidural or nothing. The anesthesiologist took a long time to come. She was an attractive woman, way too well-groomed to be a person who stabs you in the back. I showed her my back. I needed to hold completely still so she could find the exact spot, which was no easy task. I knew all too well: an error in precision and I could end up paralyzed. She finally found what she was looking for and she stuck me. Two more contractions and the pain ceased. It was a relief. We grew so relaxed that J started taking photos and videos of me in which I pretended I was in pain. I posed while miming fake screams. Who would know? It would be the false version of my authentic suffering. I was in a kind of limbo, the Disneyland of labor. It made me laugh so hard to not be in pain that I peed on myself and, since I was anesthetized, I didn't even realize it. Not until the nurse came in and dried me off.

From that point on everything is a little foggy. I remember that a doctor came in to tell me that the epidural had slowed my progress and that they were going to give me the famous "oxytocin drip." Oxytocin, from the Greek for "rapid birth," is the hormone that stimulates contractions, make them more intense and triggers birth. I refused. Presumably, a woman produces this hormone naturally, but the anesthesia had blocked its production. The doctor came back, this time accompanied by the friendly midwife, to tell me that they needed to rupture my membranes because my labor was progressing very slowly and we needed to speed things up. I was still at five centimeters. I refused. The doctor insisted. He told me it was necessary. That labor had stalled and it was now dangerous. The doctor was in a hurry. Maybe he had an important dinner to get to.

I knew I'd lost the battle, that my labor was no longer my own. I had failed. The voices in my head finally fell silent.

And all the prophecies were confirmed: what begins with a cry for an epidural almost always ends with an induced labor. But not because, as the horrible midwife had suggested, the majority of pregnant women are, deep down, a bunch of cowards incapable of making it to the finish line on our own.

It's simply that a hospital, even in a special room and with a gigantic ball, is not exactly a relaxing place.

Before making it into this room, I was sent home once and again, obliged to pay for, and put up with, two taxis, to call an ambulance, and suffer repeated mistreatment from the Emergency Department staff. When I found the person who could help me she left to attend to other women. By the time I reached my destination, I was already exhausted and wracked by pain and I could find nothing that might have allowed me to ground myself in what was happening to me. I'm not trying to justify myself; maybe I could have been less ambivalent in my preparations for the birth and also more radical. Maybe I should have been more firm with the doctors. But doing it a different way didn't guarantee that I'd have my dream birth either. I know because all of my friends have had births that didn't go according to plan. Aixi, who had gone to a cabin in the countryside to give birth, had spent two days and nights in labor and, badly dehydrated, had to rush to a clinic to get an IV because she was on the verge of fainting from hunger and exhaustion and didn't have the strength to push. Irene, the most pro-natural of us all, had ended up having a dreaded C-section. Anything could happen. There was too much noise all around me to hear what my body might be saying. All I could hear was its screams.

The doctor inserted a hook and ruptured my membranes, allowing the amniotic fluid to come out. My water was broken. A routine procedure. An hour later they came back to monitor me and concluded that I still wasn't ripe and they needed to give me the oxytocin. A medicalized birth, from A to Z. After the drip, the most savage of the contractions returned and I almost asked them to top off my epidural.

What begins in an ambulance always ends like this.

Now I'm on the bed in the delivery room. I think that's J dressed in green like just one more of the attendants filling the room. There are about ten people in there. As far as I know, not one of them bought a ticket to see the show. They're all encouraging me at once. Two women stand very close to me. I trust them; I have an urgent need to trust someone. They say positive things to me, give technical guidance, tell me to breathe, to push, to breathe. J holds my hand, I look at him with pleading eyes, he tells me I'm doing great. He's transparent; I know he's making a supreme effort to appear calm, but you can see how nervous he is by the way his Adam's apple moves in his long neck when he swallows. He strokes my forehead with a damp hand and our cold sweat intermingles. I don't stop looking at his beautiful eyes, I see myself through him because it's preferable to seeing myself through my own, relentlessly ruthless gaze. I look at him and I believe that everything is under control. This is an essential part of our life together. I know that he's worried about me, that he doesn't want me to suffer or for anything bad to happen to me. Up until now it's been the two of us; we take care of each other, we have each other's backs. But in just a few minutes this is all going to change. He looks at me and he looks down there, the door our daughter will come through. He doesn't go away, he doesn't let me go, he doesn't let me fall. The midwife calls to him to take a look and see how close we are. They can see her now. I wish there were a mirror. I hate that I can't bend over to see it from their perspective and that, instead, they have to tell me about it. J tells me that he can see her, that he can see her head. They tell me to give one last enormous push. My only triumph has been that the midwife has agreed to hold off on an episiotomy for as long as possible, and in the end, it won't be necessary. A woman talks me through it. I push with all my might, but she doesn't come out. I tear slightly. I'll need two stitches that will heal quickly; more bogeymen banished. The midwife narrates the whole thing like it's a soccer match. Time to breathe and push again. Everyone congratulates me for the slightest progress but I don't pay them any mind. For the first time in my life, I'm focused on something other than just myself. I try harder than ever, I turn red, I sweat, I open. Next to me, the monitor shows my baby's heart rate. I look at the fluctuations of her fragile life, which depends on me doing things right. Everything will be like that from now on. I think I'm going to be overcome by emotion and, as always, I want to avoid that at all costs. And, as always, I will fail. She's coming now, she's making her way, I can feel her coming, I see her, held aloft, smeared with fluids from my womb, warm, discolored, with the face of a boxer. They show her to me like a waiter shows you a bottle of wine, as if I could say that I don't want her. They lay her on top of me. She's no longer an extension of me. She's another. Will I cry? If I ask myself this question it means I will not cry.

EPILOGUE

ROOM 525. Flowers. Recognition.

Her skin is like that of an aquatic being. It seems like I might find a piece of seaweed between her toes at any moment. I'm back to marine metaphors, and so what?

She's in one piece. All she has is a spot on one eye. A battle wound. She smells like something very clean. She is very small, thin, and pale. Her hands are very long and translucent like a vampire's. Her hair is black, damp, and greasy. Her eyes are narrow and wide-set. They are two slits that open like E.T.'s eyes. I think it's because she's afraid; a little more than I am.

Looking at your newborn baby is like being on ecstasy. A combination of extreme tenderness, apprehension, and the urge to dance.

Every time she comes back from being examined she looks frightened. I need to get out of here as soon as possible. I hate everyone. I want to murder the nurses, the families, and the other babies.

The woman sharing my room has asked for a fourth bottle for her baby. She says the boy is hungry and she doesn't have enough milk. And, in fact, he doesn't stop crying. Her husband hasn't come to see her today. She calls him on the phone and they argue. I'm afraid that he's out celebrating the birth of his son with his friends. She hangs up on him. The brand-new mother turns on the television. She watches trash TV. Next to this woman, I'm Miss Universe.

My dark breast is a wellspring. It's solace for every ill, it takes away hunger and fear. I always knew this. My body is perfect for this. I marvel at her tiny mouth latching onto my nipple. I can't believe she likes it.

A nurse comes in and says she's going to show us how to give a baby a massage. Of course, she hasn't brought in a baby doll for such a purpose, so she takes my roommate's actual baby and smears him with cream, massaging him here and there as she explains the entire process with utter indifference. The baby cries desperately. I tell her to stop, that I don't care about learning more. This makes the nurse angry.

"Galant the elephant and Leo the mosquito live on the banks of a stream in a house that is green. There they grow tangerines and never never cause a scene." I know lots of children's songs. I just realized this. What a huge bonus.

From a poem I wrote over a decade ago (I don't know why):
My peace was a lie / mama lay me down to sleep in full daylight / in her yellow house she hid / the courtyards of the night / she closed my eyes with doll's pins / she believed in this manner of protection / but she never warned me of the danger / kick, deserted park, bald tree / now I rock in your small hands / and I see you and I try to sing some true song / do not fall asleep, little one, to these melodies / wake up if you hear / today or tomorrow / the lullaby.

I'm carrying Lena in my arms. J is taking care of the final discharge paperwork. I'm waiting for him very near the door. Outside it is a glorious summer day. The sun is shining. Suddenly, a woman approaches me. She is probably Filipina. I don't understand everything she's saying. She wants to see my baby, please, just for a minute. I show Lena to her. She tells me I have a very pretty baby. Her eyes brim with tears. I ask her what's wrong. I try to comfort her. I don't know what's happening. She asks me when my baby was born, if everything went well. I tell her yes, thank you. Fear invades me and I hug Lena tightly. I start to think that, at any moment, this woman is going to snatch her from me and run away with her. She's surely a psychopath. This is how the sweet story of a pregnant woman ends these days. Her newborn kidnapped at the door to the maternity ward. The story becomes a crime story. I move away from her, looking for J. He's noticed what's happening; I walk toward him, he walks toward me, but the Filipina is following behind me, she wants to explain something to me. She catches up with me, tells me that she also had a baby and he looked just like my baby, but he died, just a few days ago, in this hospital, everything was fine when he was born and then they told her he had died, and now it had been several days and they still hadn't given her his tiny corpse. I feel dizzy. I tell her I'm sorry; it's all I can do. "Is it a boy?" she asks me, sobbing. I tell her no, it's a girl. "Mine was a boy," she says. J gets me out of there. I hear the woman shouting after me that I should take very good care of my baby girl.

———

We're hiding in a closet. "Daddy, come here!" Lena shouts. We look at each other in the darkness. Shhhhhh. We don't make any noise. When I was little, I loved hiding in closets. There was a huge one with a sliding door in my grandmother's house. The scent of mothballs, the hanging clothes brushing against my face, holding completely still, listening to the sounds outside and waiting for someone to find me or at least to look for me. Here comes Daddy. We crouch down. We're ready to scare him.

Lena prepares a plate of dry leaves, twigs, and raw noodles. Now she's the one who feeds me. She raises her small spoon and feeds me invisible bites that taste delicious. She tells me her baby pooped and she puts one of her own diapers on him. Then she puts him in a little stroller, slings a bag over her shoulder, and waves goodbye.

AFTERWORD

DEAR COCO AND AMARU,

It's been ten years since I published *Nine Moons*, the book in which I recounted the nine months I spent with you, Coco, inside of me. A lot of things have changed since then and there are some things that, unfortunately, never change. Among the things that have changed is the fact that we are no longer a family made up of a mom, dad, and daughter, as we were back then. Now we are three "adres," as you call us, and you have a little brother I did not give birth to. From the beginning, to our great delight, you've been an accomplice, embracing the change, adapting quickly and expressing pride in your new polyamorous family.

You're thirteen years old now, Coco, but you still haven't wanted to read the book about your nine months in utero. You always say, with your customary dark humor, why would you want to read it when you already lived it? Well, to be precise, I did read the last chapter to you out loud once and you laughed your head off, especially at the part about how you were nearly kidnapped at the front door of the hospital. We also still wonder together what might have become of that mother who saw her lost baby in you, and it makes us both feel sad.

When they told me you were a girl, I wrote you a letter, not unlike the one I'm writing you today, now that you've told me you aren't exactly a girl. A few months ago, you told us that you are trans nonbinary, that your name is Coco and that the name your dad and I gave you when you were born, a decision we agonized over, is now your deadname.

It's funny to reread that letter in which I confess to you that, during the first four months of gestation, I had referred to you in the masculine and after the ultrasound it was hard for me to suddenly start using the feminine, like when a friend changes sexes. And now it's happened again. In some way, you've been born a second time, this time for yourself. The pronoun you've asked us to use for you is *elle*. Your bedroom is covered in gay pride flags. The other day, we went out to eat and you asked me a lot of questions about sex. You're at that age. That day we felt more mother and *hije* than ever.

You became radicalized some time ago. You put yourself out there, more than I ever did at your age, and that's exactly why I'm not afraid. I would be afraid if you'd never told me who you are, and then I'd be afraid of myself. You know? Sometimes I think that those right-wing extremists are afraid of their children because their children represent change, transformation, renovation, everything that scares them. Those sorts of people never change. They can't imagine how powerfully emotional it is to see these people who came out of us, but who belong only to themselves, fully living out who they are.

Every day you listen, indignant, to politicians promoting laws that would make it so that children are not taught to differentiate between consensual sex and sexual abuse, like, for example, when they are touched by a priest or their own father. Politicians who are also against the sex education and birth control that help prevent teen pregnancy and unsafe abortions, which kill so many young women in the country where I was born and in other places around the world where abortion is illegal and where those who dare to seek one are persecuted. You know that the ultraright is harassing and censoring your teachers. I laugh when you tell me about your classmate who calls you a feminazi and how, as a Secret Santa gift at Christmas, you gave him a Spanish flag on which you had written "legal and free abortions, xo," but deep down, I'm not really laughing that hard.

It's true that we "ideologized" you to fight for equality, for your rights, for your freedom. And your friend, the one who calls you feminazi, was ideologized to attack these things. And yet, in theory, you both go to the public school to be educated according to the Universal Declaration of Human Rights, and that is what we are going to defend together. Because that other friend of yours who is still to terrified to tell their mother that they're not a girl goes to school there, too. But you always call them by their true name. And that's why I love you.

Amaru, *bebé*, you didn't know the old world, you came straight into the new one, or, more accurately, you revolutionized it and pushed us from theory into practice, from dream into action. When they tried to stop us because there were "too many of us," the three of us, your father and your two mothers, more or less forced our way into the doctor's office for the ultrasound so we could see you swimming in amniotic fluid and listen to the beating of the heart that would bring us the latest news. Roci gave birth to you at home and Jaime and I were there to greet you. We gave you my last name as your middle name, Amaru Wiener, while we work to one day change the laws so that, as the child of all three of us, you can have all three of our names as your last name.

Sometimes I ask myself what sort of a mother I am to you. You know perfectly well that Laura, the little girl in your book, has only one mommy and that I pretend every night that she goes to the supermarket with her two mommies, but you let me. What you like is to crack up when Laura wants to do everything on her own, put the green apples in the bag and push the shopping cart that's twice her size, because you do the same thing. There's another book you like a lot, *A Mother's Heart*, about a mother and a child. It tells about how there's a very fine, almost invisible thread that connects a mother's heart to her child's heart, and so everything that happens to the child also happens to the mother: her heart dances when the child laughs or contracts when the child is sick or feels sad. I don't change that one because it's too beautiful, and although it speaks of just one mother, I know that when I read it to you, you know that it tells the story of my heart, and that when Roci reads it to you, it tells the story of hers. When I finish reading it, you always pretend to be a baby kitten, you want to grab my breast and lick my face.

Do you remember when, the other day, our friend asked you who your favorite character was from Paw Patrol and you said it was Ryder and then Chase and then, in the end, you didn't know how to answer? Well, don't worry, you don't have to have favorites, or compare the things you like. It's enough that there's room inside you for all of them. Don't think I'm only saying this to you; I'm saying it to myself as well because sometimes I forget. For example, the other day, after you fell down you went running to Roci and someone commented: "There's only one mother!"

The other day in the park a little boy told you that his father had gone on a trip and you said: "Well, I have two mommies." Simple as that: some people have a dad who's gone on a trip and other people have two mommies. Easy to understand. I like to think that you came not out of my body but out of my imagination, that I'm nursing you with the colostrum of my dreams. When I took my first good long look at you, I saw in your face all the faces of those I love, except my own. But now, when we crack up laughing at the use and abuse in our vocabulary of the word "poto"—which is a much more fun and tender and Peruvian way of saying "butt"—when you change the words to boring songs and stories, when you change my world, our world, I see myself, I see us in your little *poto* face.

—FEBRUARY, 2020

ACKNOWLEDGMENTS

To Elsi Bravo, for not telling me everything and allowing me to tell it in my own way. To Elisa, for playing the mom and the daughter. To Vilma Zavaleta, for her hero's heart. To Jessica and Patty Bravo, for doing my makeup in the bathroom of their house on Mello Franco. To Karina Rodríguez, ultrawarrior. To Adriana, our firefly.

To Claudio López de Lamadrid, for adopting me. To Sergio Vilela, for his sweet expectation. To María Lynch, fallen from heaven. To Diego Salazar, without whose advice this book would not have been written. To Toño Angulo, for the final title. To Javier Calvo for touching me with his wizard's wand. To Mónica Carmona, Sofía Lecumberri, Marta Borrell, Eva Cuenca, and Marta Díaz for their care with this manuscript.

To the mothers all around me, to those who have yet to become mothers and to those who never will. To Victoria Castillo and Elena Fresco. To Aunt Julia and Aunt Bertha. To Elena Ramos, María Esther Mesía, Chela Ulloa, and

Inés Agressot. To Nélida Céspedes and Teresa Carpio. To my mother-friends: Micaela Ameri, Inés Velarde, Vania Portugal, Regina Cortés, Ima Garmendia, Tati Quiñones, Maribel Tovar, Victoria Bautista, Marcela Robles, Carmen Pérez de Vega, Carmen Olivas, Ale Barba, Mónica Arrese, Malú Ponte, Isa Sánchez, Mara Lethem, Bea Fluxá, Ximena Urbina, Mónica Escudero. To all of them for confiding in me about their nine moons and more.

To Alejandra, Melisa, Valeria, Romina, Mateo, Micaelita, Adriana (x 2), Bárbara, Lucía, Alaia, Max, Sol, Octavio, Adriano, Mauricio, Joaquín, Oliver, Paulo (x 2), Claudia, Judit, Berta, Elvis, Gael, and Maiku, for changing everything.

To Jaime Rodríguez and to Lena Rodríguez Wiener, my wild bunch.

ABOUT THE AUTHOR
AND TRANSLATOR

GABRIELA WIENER (Lima, 1975) is the acclaimed author six collections of *crónicas*, including *Sexographies* (2018), her first to be translated into English. She writes regularly for the newspapers *El País* (Spain), *La República* (Peru), and others in the US and Europe. In Madrid, she worked as editor of the Spanish edition of *Marie Claire*. She lives in Madrid.

JESSICA POWELL has published dozens of translations of literary works by a wide variety of Latin American writers, including Silvina Ocampo, Pablo Neruda and Antonio Benítez Rojo. She is the recipient of a National Endowment for the Arts Translation Fellowship and has been a finalist for the Best Translated Book Award and longlisted for the National Translation Award. She lives in Santa Barbara.